# SCHEIN'S COMMON SENSE WOUND Care Management



**Moshe Schein MD FACS**

tfm Publishing Limited, Castle Hill Barns, Harley, Nr Shrewsbury, SY5 6LX, UK
Tel: +44 (0)1952 510061; Fax: +44 (0)1952 510192
E-mail: info@tfmpublishing.com; Web site: www.tfmpublishing.com

Editing, Design & Typesetting: Nikki Bramhill BSc (Hons) Dip Law
First edition: © July 2026
Cartoons: © 2026 Evgeniy E. (Perya) Perelygin, MD
Front cover painting: © 2026 Dan Schein (E-mail: danschein@gmail.com)

Paperback ISBN: 978-1-913755-73-7

E-book editions: © 2026
ePub ISBN: 978-1-913755-74-4
Web pdf ISBN: 978-1-913755-75-1
ePub (accessible) ISBN: 978-1-913755-76-8



Printed by Gutenberg Press Ltd., Gudja Road, Tarxien, GXQ 2902, Malta
Tel: +356 2398 2201; Fax: +356 2398 2290
E-mail: info@gutenberg.com.mt; Web site: www.gutenberg.com.mt

# Contents

**Preface** v

**Acknowledgements** vi

PART I — The basics 1

**Chapter 1** 3
The wound care industry

**Chapter 2** 9
The 'problem wounds' — the wounds you will see in the wound clinic

**Chapter 3** 21
Wound healing and non-healing — why are these wounds 'problematic'?

**Chapter 4** 29
Assessment of the patients and their wounds

PART II — General concepts of wound management 45

**Chapter 5** 47
Wound debridement

**Chapter 6** 55
Contamination, colonization, and infection

**Chapter 7** 75
Dressings

**Chapter 8** 85
Compression

**Chapter 9** 97
Negative pressure wound therapy (NPWT) or VAC (vacuum-assisted closure)

**Chapter 10** 105
Palliative care

**Chapter 11** 111
Prevention

**Chapter 12** 115
Gimmicks

**PART III — Specific wounds** 119

**Chapter 13** 121
Venous ulcers

**Chapter 14** 127
Diabetic ulcers

**Chapter 15** 137
Ischemic ulcers

**Chapter 16** 145
Pressure ulcers

**Chapter 17** 153
Post-surgical wounds

**Chapter 18** 155
Post-traumatic wounds and hematomas

**Chapter 19** 165
Morbid obesity-related wounds

**Chapter 20** 169
Miscellaneous wounds

**Epilogue** 171

**Index** 173

# Preface

After practicing general surgery for more than 45 years, I felt my age creeping up on me. What are the options for an old surgeon, I asked myself, before 'senility' steps in? Some useless administrative position? Full-time scrub assistant to younger colleagues? Retirement? **But then I thought: why not wound care?**

Looking around, I noticed how the 'wound care industry' is mushrooming around the country and our communities; I observed old patients who must travel for hours to one of the various 'wound care clinics' where nurses, or nurse practitioners are providing the so-called 'modern dedicated wound care', being supervised, closely or not so closely, by some semi-retired physicians. So, I thought, why not provide expert wound care to those poor souls, closer to their homes? **Why not establish a local wound care clinic combined with my general surgery practice? Who understands wounds more than a general surgeon!?**

**Like most surgeons, I considered myself an expert in wound care.** After all, surgeons do nothing but produce wounds and then heal them. To us, it seems so simple: we cut, we suture, it heals. Sure, some wounds do not heal promptly or get infected; so, we remove the sutures, give some antibiotics, sometimes we must debride or suture again; occasionally a drain is required, maybe a 'wound VAC'. Oh yes, some wounds go on smoldering but are lost to follow-up and turn up elsewhere, for example, with an infected mesh needing removal by another surgeon...

As to the actual wound management, I always preached that we don't need anything fancy. We irrigate the wound with the solution *d'jour*, based on local tastes and dogmas. We cover it with some gauze, a bandage, and tape — sometimes even some elaborate dressing. Eventually, nature accomplishes what it should, and sooner or later, most wounds we inflict do heal. I believed that most wounds do not need to be cultured and that antibiotics are hugely overused. (I still believe it...)

But my perspective changed gradually as I established my own wound care clinic and thus joined the 'wound care industry'. **Very soon, I realized that the wounds seen in a dedicated wound care clinic are different!**

**So what does an old surgeon, now a wound care specialist, do? Writes another book!**

# Acknowledgements

I wish to express my gratitude to the following friends for their 'indirect' contribution to this book:

To Stephanie Bixler, NP, a superb wound care specialist, a role model and mentor;

To Dr. Subramanian Natarajan for encouraging me to incorporate 'wound care' into my general surgery practice;

To my manager Heather Repka for all her support;

To my colleagues Dr. Bill Krause, Dr. Katie Winiarczyk, Kellsey Fellbaum, NP, and Brita Bush, NP, for their help with patient care.

And to my dedicated and tireless assistant, Carla Egle — I couldn't have developed and maintained the wound care clinic without her.

# PART I

## The basics

# Chapter 1

## The wound care industry

*I dressed him and God healed him.*

**Ambroise Paré, 1510–1590**

### The wound care industry

There are more than 2000 specialized wound care clinics in the USA — many attached to hospitals and clinics, but some are in private practices, exclusively focused on wound care. It seems that a wide range of specialties have jumped on the **lucrative bandwagon** — plastic, vascular, podiatry, dermatology, physiotherapy — focusing on wound care within their practices. People from all sorts of medical and quasi-medical backgrounds attend one of the many 'wound care courses', pass some 'certifying examination', and with the fresh diploma on the wall, they become 'wound care experts', some of them offering 'voodoo'-type care (■ Figure 1.1).

Talking to my surgical colleagues across the world, I hear that the situation is not that much different in most countries. Dr. Mathias Kalkum of Germany summarized the situation aptly.

"In Germany, it is not much different from Mexico or the US. If there is money in it, somebody cares; if not, it is left to the nurses and a plethora of expensive dressings. But the truth is, it needs somebody who knows. Who knows that healing requires oxygen, which requires perfusion. Who knows how to palpate for a pulse. Who knows when or how to take a swab. Who knows that bacterial growth is not the same as infection, and that not every 'inflammation' needs antibiotics. And someone who knows how and what to teach the nurses and when it is best to listen to them."

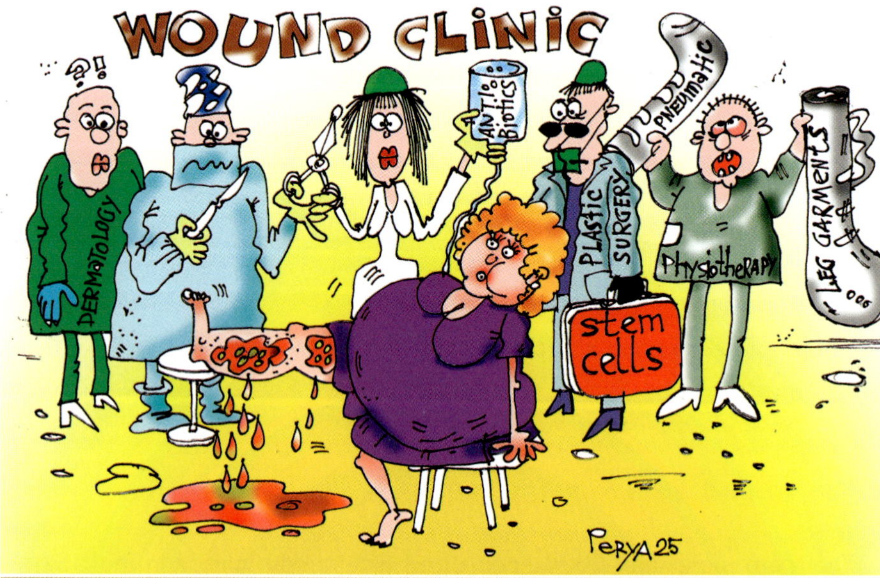


Figure 1.1. The wound care clinic.

**Undoubtedly, 'modern' wound care worldwide is chaotic. In this little book, I will attempt to apply some common sense to that chaos.**

Wound care is immensely costly. According to the Centers for Medicare and Medicaid Services (CMS), the estimated cost of wound care in the USA for 1 year (2023) was **$117 billion**, averaging $13,355 dollars per patient. Search online or walk around the supermarkets, and you will note the vast spectrum of wound care products offered; then you will understand why the wound care product market has been estimated to range between 22 and 33 billion US $. (I promise not to bore you too much with figures and statistics.)

As always, where there is money to be made, the industry comes in. **The more older, fatter, and sicker our population becomes, the more complex wounds they develop, the larger and more lucrative the wound care market becomes.**

Hospitals, clinics, home care agencies, nursing homes and, of course, product manufacturers all join in to exploit the demand. Add to it the 'parasites', like the companies serving as intermediaries — companies that receive orders for wound care products from the 'providers', arrange for approval from the insurance companies, and ship the products to the patients' homes.

## Establishing a 'wound care clinic'

So, after taking an online course and passing a 'wound care certifying examination', I visited, together with my medical assistant (MA), a few established wound care clinics, shadowing trusted 'wound care experts' — and then I opened my own wound care clinic. To do so, you need the following:

- **A dedicated assistant**. This can be a nurse, an MA, whatever — someone who learns from you the wound care 'routine', who knows how to order, store, and rapidly assess the vast paraphernalia needed.
- **Storage space**. For the broad spectrum of 'products' that must be readily accessible.
- **Support team**. These patients are complex! From time to time you need to refer to (or talk with) a podiatrist (the feet are the location of most 'problem wounds'), a vascular surgeon (for 'ischemic wounds'), home care agencies (to continue wound care at home), social services (many of such patients are indigent or 'neglected'), infection disease specialists (you should listen to them but not always agree with their recommendations), occupational therapists (some know how to combat lymphedema) and, of course, the patients' primary care providers (to help you improve the patients' general condition).
- **Patience. You will need lots of patience — patience and serenity for the patients (most of them afflicted with multiple comorbidities) and patience and endurance for their wounds**. While surgical, traumatic, or pressure wounds can develop instantly or within a few days, their healing requires many weeks, months, or even years. **Some wounds will never heal** — here your task is to 'maintain' the wounds, preventing deterioration and helping the patient to 'live with his wound' until nature takes its course. You may need to attend to some wounds regularly for years!
- **Fitness and endurance**. Of course, you could direct wound care management from your office, looking at images on your laptop and instructing your disciples on how to treat the wounds. But if you wish to be an active player in the 'wound care game', you need to be physically fit and agile. Many of those patients have limited mobility.

Commonly, we find ourselves lying on the floor to debride and dress their wounds (■ Figure 1.2).

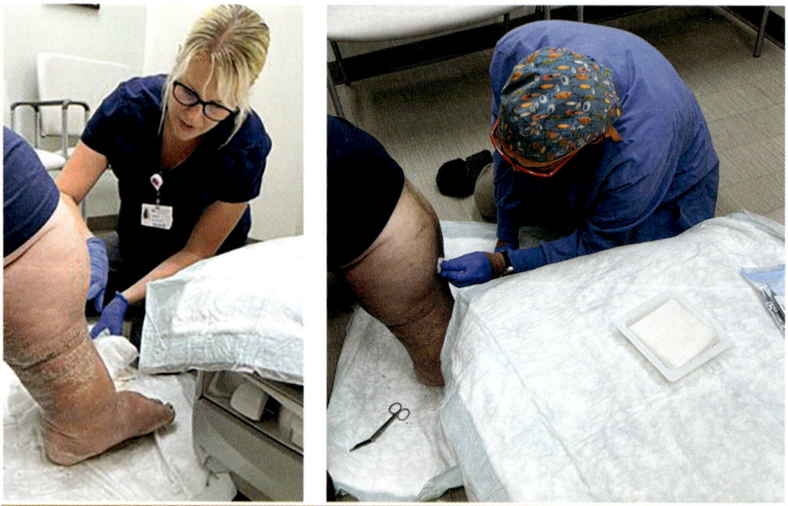

**Figure 1.2. Be ready to lay on the floor. The author and Carla, his assistant.**

## What is this book all about?

**To the novice, wound care is confusing**: so many options are advocated to achieve the same goal, so many expert opinions, so many products pushed on you. **In this slim book (call it a 'monograph'), I have tried to alleviate some of that confusion by offering a concise, straightforward approach to wound care — based on established principles and common sense — with as little BS as possible**.

Here, you won't hear much about the physiology of wound healing (or non-healing), and I won't burden you with obscure figures or unreliable statistics. I know you might be overwhelmed by the wide range of wound care products available, so I will simplify the topic as well, mentioning only a few brand names as examples. **And like in our other books in the 'series' of *Schein's Common Sense*..., I won't be citing any references from the literature!**

**You may ask, 'Why? Where is the 'scientific evidence?' But the truth of the matter is that the science of wound care is flawed**.

**Asking one of the AI machines about the 'quality of wound care studies', you will get a response like this:**

"The quality of evidence in wound care studies has historically been mixed, **often falling short of the rigor seen in other medical fields**. Several challenges contribute to this:

- **Heterogeneity of wounds**: chronic wounds vary widely in etiology, size, location, and patient comorbidities, making standardization difficult.
- **Lack of standardized outcomes**: studies often use inconsistent definitions of healing, timeframes, and endpoints, which hampers comparison and meta-analysis.
- **Methodological limitations**: many studies are small, lack blinding, or use surrogate endpoints. Randomized controlled trials (RCTs), while possible, are underutilized due to logistical and ethical complexities."

**Significantly, most such studies, advocating yet another 'wonder cure' for wounds, are supported by the industry**. Did you ever look at which countries most of such studies are reported from? China and India are primary sources. How does it work? The producer of the 'wonder product' calls some obscure Chinese University, tells them what results he needs… and *voilà* — the data and results are manufactured. So, when I see enthusiastic wound care 'specialists' using some novel biological material (costing a few thousand bucks), desperately trying to heal a wound which will never heal, in a limb which is going to be amputated a few months later — I roll my eyes with disgust.

**Talking about AI**: these days, each of you could produce a similar book to this one in a few hours. Just enter each of this book's chapter titles into a robust AI machine and ask: 'Please write a chapter of 3000 words on this topic', and in a few seconds you will get a beautifully formatted manuscript including references. But, of course, the AI product is based on the available literature, the flawed literature — it doesn't weed out useless data. **It cannot offer wisdom backed by principles and experience — and that is precisely what this book is offering you.**

**When I write in the following chapters that a particular product or method lacks credible evidence, I base such opinion on an in-depth review of the available data. If you don't trust me, you can dig into the 'literature' yourself…**

**"The discipline of wound care, compared with most other disciplines and specialties, is basically the 'Wild Wild West' of patient care."**

# Chapter 2

## The 'problem wounds' — the wounds you will see in the wound clinic

*In politically incorrect terms, the wound care clinic represents a 'cesspool', into which other specialties dump patients with wounds that they cannot (or do not want) to deal with* (■ Figure 2.1).

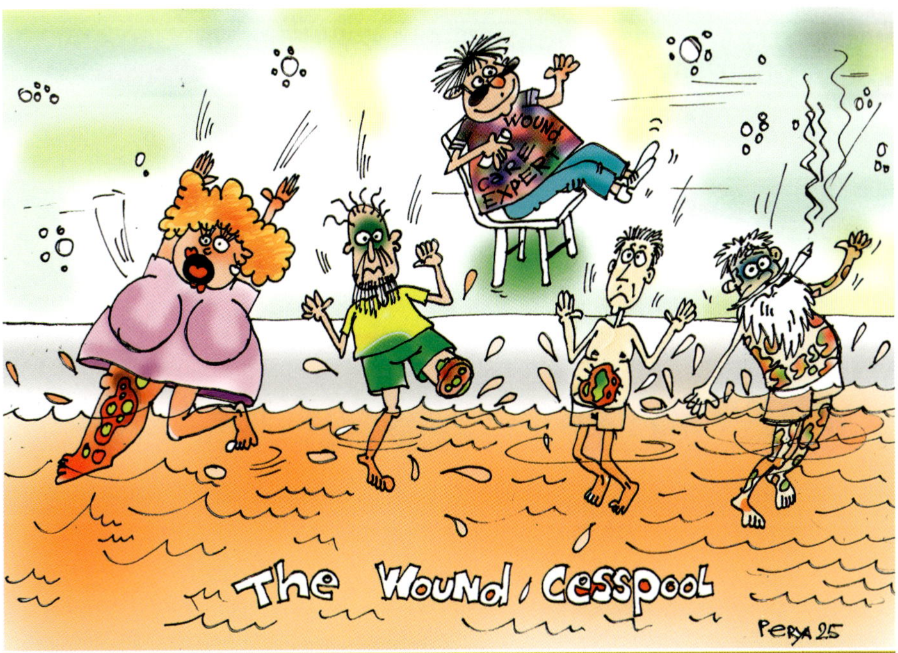


**Figure 2.1. The wound 'cesspool'.**

**A 'typical wound care clinic patient'**: think about a super obese giantess with legs like elephants, with horrendous ulcers, against the background of venous stasis and lymphedema — oozing and soaking her stinking dressings; her diabetes uncontrolled, despite all efforts by her primary care provider. Her husband cannot cope with the need to change his wife's dressings twice a day — he is morbidly obese as well. They are desperate! The patient presents to various emergency rooms, receiving various ointments and a few courses of antibiotics, until someone refers her to your wound care clinic for 'debridement' of infected ulcers. **So, how would you treat this patient? Now it's your turn — you can't dump her.**

**Dedicated wound care clinics exist to treat these types of chronic or acute-on-chronic wounds that are so common in our aging and sicker populations.**

■ **Table 2.1 lists the main groups of wounds in random order.** The proportion of each group that you will see depends on your specific environment. How to assess and diagnose each group is discussed in ➲ Chapter 4. Each of these entities has been the subject of entire books and numerous publications. I expect you did, or will do, some additional reading... or YouTube watching.

| **Table 2.1. Types of wounds seen in the wound care clinic (many will be of mixed etiology.** |
| --- |
| ■ Venous/stasis ulcers. |
| ■ Diabetic ulcers. |
| ■ Ischemic ulcers. |
| ■ Pressure/decubitus ulcers. |
| ■ Post-surgical wounds. |
| ■ Post-traumatic wounds and hematomas. |
| ■ Morbid obesity-related wounds. |
| ■ Miscellaneous. |

## Venous/stasis ulcers (see ➲ Chapter 13)

**These ulcers occur due to valve failure in the leg veins, leading to venous hypertension**. The underlying causes are neglected, longstanding **primary varicose veins** or previous episodes of deep venous thrombosis (**post-phlebitis syndrome**). **Obesity is a common associated factor.**

Typically, they are located against the background of longstanding stasis dermatitis on the medial lower leg, especially near the medial malleolus, but can also develop higher on the shin (■ Figure 2.2). **Note: most of the venous ulcers you will see are not typical (the 'typical' ulcers can be easily managed in the primary care set-up). Instead, they will belong to the 'mixed' category (see below).**

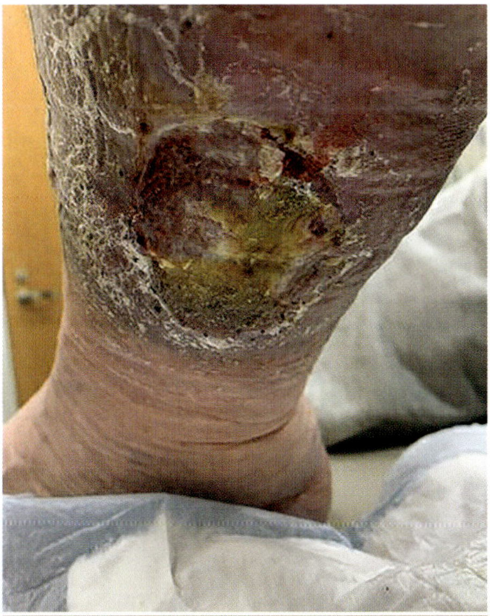

**Figure 2.2. A venous leg ulcer developing against the background of stasis dermatitis.**

## Diabetic ulcers (see ➲ Chapter 14)

**Diabetic ulcers are chronic wounds that commonly develop on the feet and toes of diabetic patients due to a combination of factors**:

- **Peripheral neuropathy**: resulting in loss of protective sensation — patients do not appreciate minor injuries to their feet. It also leads to muscle weakness, causing foot deformities that, in turn, create new pressure points — prone to callus formation and ulcers.
- **Peripheral vascular disease (PVD)**: involving small- and/or medium-sized vessels, is commonly present and results in tissue ischemia.
- **Metabolic dysfunction and immune deficiency**: hyperglycemia due to poor glycemic control impairs wound healing, exposes ulcers to infection, and impairs their treatment.

**Again, many of such ulcers are 'mixed'**: the product of **diabetes**, repeated **trauma** and/or **pressure** wounds, in **obese** patients, with **PVD**, who suffer from **varicose veins** or had **DVT** in the past. **A perfect storm!**

## Ischemic ulcers (➲ Chapter 15)

**'Pure' ischemic ulcers, which occur when tissues are deprived of blood supply, develop typically in the lower limbs** — especially the feet, toes, and ankles. Suggestive history (e.g. atherosclerosis, smoking, claudication) is not always present, as the cause of ischemia could be embolic (e.g. 'blue toe syndrome'). **Of course, many of the ischemic wounds you will see are 'mixed'**, associated with diabetes, trauma, obesity, and/or developing postoperatively (e.g. the foot or leg amputation site fails to heal because of persistent ischemia).

## Pressure/decubitus ulcers (➲ Chapter 16)

**Pressure ulcers (also called decubitus ulcers or bedsores) are injuries to the skin and underlying tissue caused by sustained pressure that reduces blood flow to the compressed areas**. It develops in people with limited mobility (confined to bed or a wheelchair). **Another mechanism** involved is **shear force**, which occurs when the skin and underlying structures move in opposing directions when the patient slides on his or her bed or wheelchair. **Excessive moisture** from leaking urine or feces, leading to tissue maceration, is a contributing factor. Many of these patients are debilitated and suffer from comorbidities, making these ulcers 'mixed' as well.

## Post-surgical wounds (➲ Chapter 17)

**In the good old days, which some of us old farts still remember, surgeons used to treat the wounds produced by their operations until complete healing took place**. Today, however, things have changed, concerning especially surgical subspecialties rather than general surgery. Patients undergoing orthopedic, vascular, or gynecological procedures are discharged home after a day or two, only to develop wound complications, and land in your wound care clinic.

True, many patients live remotely from the 'ivory towers' where the procedures have been performed, and they prefer to have the complications managed locally. But hey, why should the bone surgeon bother for a few months with a non-healing amputation stump when he or she has so many hips to replace; why should a vascular surgeon waste his or her time on a festering groin wound (soon the synthetic graft will be exposed) — shouldn't the time be better used with endovascular procedures? And the cardiothoracic surgeon has to focus on the heart — prolonged care of an infected sternal wound is unrewarding, whereas the commonly non-healing leg wounds at the site of vein harvesting (■ Figure 2.3) are 'beyond their scope'. **Thus, a broad spectrum of complicated postop wounds may end up in your 'cesspool'**, not only weeks or months after the index operation, but even years, as with synthetic mesh placed in an abdominal hernia, which slowly migrates to the surface of the skin.

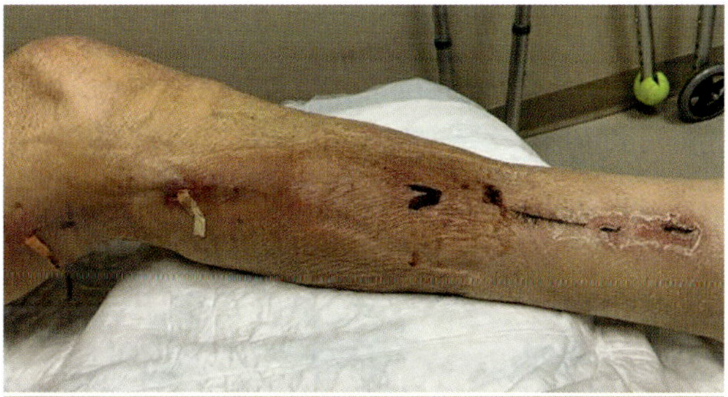

**Figure 2.3. A patient presenting a month after CABG with infected wounds at the site of saphenous vein harvesting. The vein harvesting was performed endoscopically. The resulting subcutaneous tunnel is full of pus, from the thigh to the ankle.**

## Post-traumatic wounds and hematomas (➲ Chapter 18)

**All sorts of wounds caused by various mechanisms of injury fail to heal and require your wound care services.** The reason they do not heal is described in ➲ Chapter 3. Such wounds tend to occur in susceptible individuals — the diabetic who scraped his leg, the diabetic who bumped his foot against his wheelchair — thus, also many post-traumatic wounds can be considered of a 'mixed' etiology.

**A common and frustrating sub-entity that we have to deal with is the post-traumatic hematoma.** As many elderly individuals are receiving some sort of anticoagulant drug (those who are not on warfarin or apixaban are on some form of antiplatelet agent), even a minor fall or blunt injury can produce significant soft tissue bleeding. Eventually, the bleeding is tamponaded by the adjacent structures. Still, the hematoma can continue to grow for days as local inflammation increases microcirculatory permeability and draws more fluid into the process.

**I find it frustrating because proper early management could prevent major prolonged morbidity, but this is commonly not the case.** Instead, in my experience, most emergency doctors and primary care providers — the first to address the acute problem — consider such hematomas a 'banal problem' requiring only an expectant approach, as long as they don't observe active bleeding or suspect a compartment syndrome of the injured extremity. So, they prescribe a pain killer, some would apply a loose compression sleeve, and tell the patient to go home: "elevate your leg... this should subside gradually..." **They do not even consider the need to stop the anticoagulant drug.**

I see such patients a few weeks later with a picture like this (■ Figure 2.4). What happened? Unlike 'deeper' hematomas (e.g. in the pelvis, rectus muscle, liver), soft tissue hematomas of the limbs do not absorb rapidly. Instead, they continue to grow, detaching the overlying skin from its blood supply, rendering it ischemic. **You will see an anticoagulated or excessively anticoagulated patient with a large swelling covered with necrotic skin.** You cannot start managing the patient until the anticoagulation is reversed. Healing such wounds requires a few months. **Obviously, immediate cessation of anticoagulation and referral to a general surgeon would have obviated such a disaster. All he or she must do then is to squeeze out the clot through a small incision and apply adequate compression.**

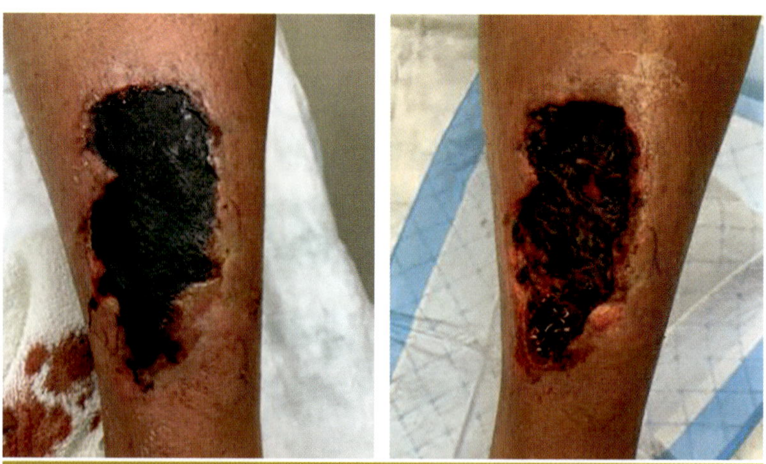

**Figure 2.4. Post-traumatic hematoma on a leg. I removed the eschar and evacuated the underlying clots, exposing a cavity and a 25 x 20cm skin defect.**

## Morbid obesity-related wounds (➲ Chapter 19)

**The current epidemic of obesity (almost a 'pandemic') afflicting the USA (and increasingly other countries) is overwhelming the wound care clinics.**

Patients with a BMI of less than 30 represent a minority — the majority consists of much heavier patients — morbid obesity with a BMI above 35 or 40; super obesity, with a BMI up to 80, is a common occurrence — we call them 'big boy' (or 'big girl') syndrome.

Like with the other wound entities listed above, legs and feet are the primary sites for wounds developing in obese patients. **It has been estimated that two-thirds of cases seen in wound care clinics involve the lower extremities!** (In some way, the practice of wound care has encroached on podiatry.) However, due to their body habitus, these patients are also prone to wounds in other body parts.

**The genesis of wounds in obese patients is multifactorial**:

- **Venous stasis: obesity causes chronically elevated intra-abdominal pressure, impairing venous return from the legs. This leads to venous hypertension that produces changes of stasis dermatitis and ulcers.** This is 'functional' venous insufficiency — the superficial veins are not damaged (no varicose veins are seen), and the deep venous system is patent (documented on ultrasound) (■ Figure 2.5).

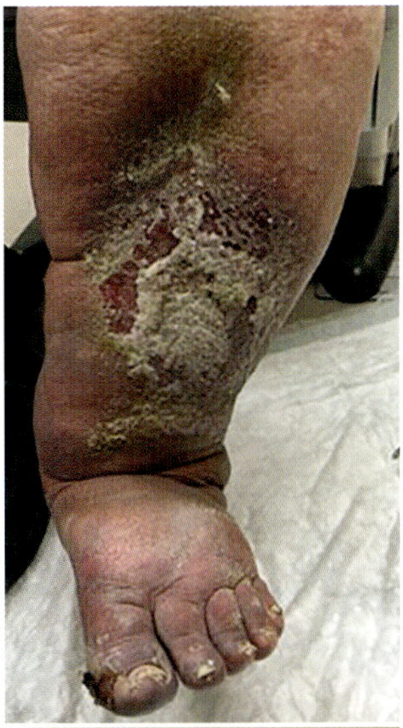

Figure 2.5. Morbidly obese (BMI 65) male patient with a typical 'stasis ulcer' on the shin.

- **Immobility and loss of the calf muscle pump**: for obvious reasons, some of these patients can hardly walk, if at all. The loss of the muscle pump, combined with prolonged sitting, leads to venous pooling in the legs, contributing to venous stasis.
- **Lymphedema**: the immense intra-abdominal pressure also impedes lymphatic drainage from the lower extremities, resulting in chronic lymphedema, which, obviously, tends to be aggravated by the commonly associated heart failure present in the morbidly obese (■ Figure 2.6).

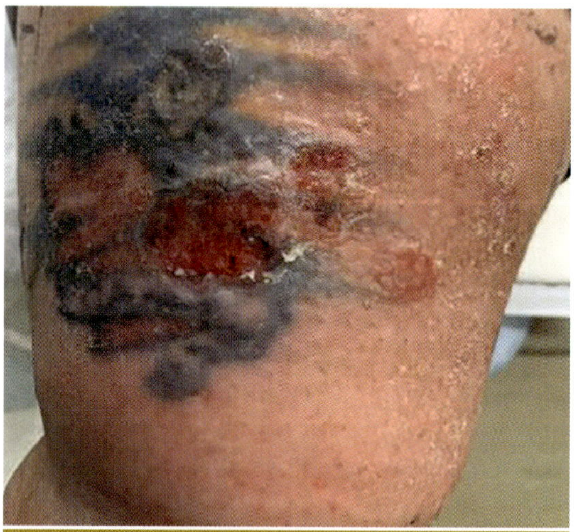

**Figure 2.6. A lady with a BMI of 79 with a fresh wound which suddenly appeared on her shin. Note the old tattoo — an area susceptible to ulceration and slows healing.**

- **Macerated skin fold**: the ample skin folds in such patients hide the deep, sunken areas from sunlight, collecting moisture, dirt, bacteria, and fungi. This leads to skin breaks and infection (■ Figure 2.7).
- **Pressure ulcers**: the combination of immobility, the heaviness and misshapenness of the trunk and limbs can result in pressure ulcers in many parts of the body (■ Figure 2.8).
- **Poor healing of adipose tissues**: poor vascularity of the fatty tissue is to blame, as is the obesity-induced chronic, low-grade inflammatory state, which impairs the immune response; add to this the commonly superimposed diabetes.
- **Nutritional deficiencies**: **paradoxically, these overfed individuals can be malnourished**. The reason is the same that makes them so

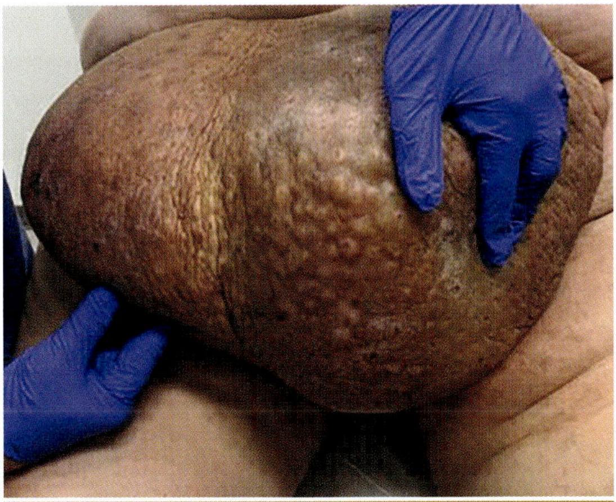

Figure 2.7. Morbidly obese (BMI 74) man. Guess what is hiding behind the pannus?

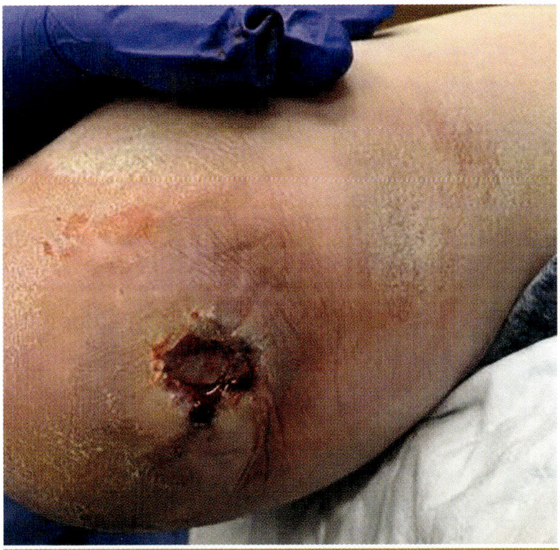

Figure 2.8. Pressure sore on the heel of a morbidly obese patient.

obese — they eat high-carbohydrate 'crap' which is poor in protein, vitamins, and other nutrients!

- **Comorbidities**: diabetes, peripheral vascular disease — you know the story…

**A condition called lipedema, affecting only women, should be mentioned in this context**. It involves symmetrical **gross accumulation of fat**

**in the column-like legs with a sudden cut-off at the ankles** ('bracelet effect'). The feet are spared. It can rarely affect the upper extremities as well. These patients are not necessarily obese. The layers of fat are tender, bruise easily, and are prone to developing wounds.

## Miscellaneous wounds (➲ Chapter 20)

**While the wound categories mentioned above represent the vast majority of patients you will see in the wound care clinic, let us not forget the 'outliers' — sporadic conditions that can produce 'problem' wounds.** The list is long; here are only a few examples:

- **Lipodermatosclerosis**: this is a chronic inflammatory condition affecting the lower legs and feet. Although chronic venous insufficiency has been implicated, varicose veins are rarely present. The subcutaneous layers are rigid (mummified), the skin hyperkeratotic and constantly desquamating. Leg and foot ulcers are common (■ Figure 2.9). Arterial supply is usually intact. **I see it in**

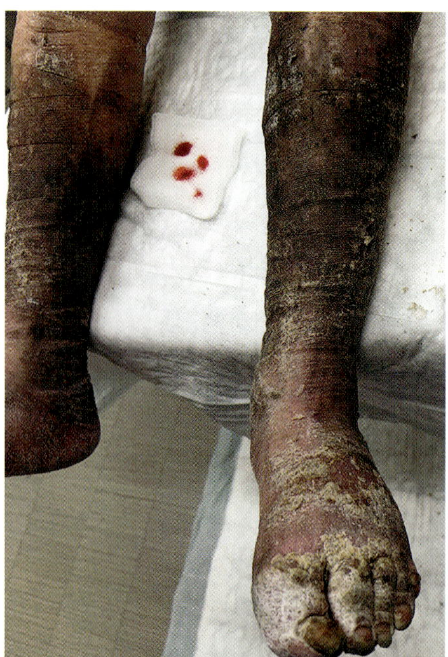

Figure 2.9. Lipodermatosclerosis in an elderly alcoholic man who smoked.

**men — the combination of prolonged smoking, drinking, and neglect commonly present in the background.**

- **Insect bites**: such as the **recluse spider**. It causes progressive cutaneous necrosis necessitating aggressive debridement.
- **Radiation therapy**: patients can present with chronic ulcers at the site of previous (excessive) irradiation even years later.
- **Pyoderma gangrenosum**: resulting in painful ulcers, typically on the legs, often associated with inflammatory bowel disease and rheumatoid arthritis. **Debridement can aggravate the condition.** Thus, as always, treating the wound without assessing the whole patient (see ➲ Chapter 4) can be dangerous!
- **Vasculitis**: small-, medium- or large-vessel vasculitis commonly affects the skin. Ulcers can develop.
- **Calciphylaxis**: painful, ischemic wounds resulting from blocking of cutaneous vessels by calcium deposits developing in patients with end-stage renal disease (diabetes and morbid obesity are additional risk factors).
- **Coumadin (warfarin)-induced skin necrosis**: acute, painful wounds occurring within a week of starting this medication, usually in areas with thick subcutaneous fat. They are caused by paradoxical clotting of subcutaneous vessels.
- **Necrobiosis lipoidica diabeticorum**: patches of discolored skin developing mostly on the shins of diabetic patients and may result in ulceration. It is often confused with stasis dermatitis.
- **Skin cancers presenting as wounds** (e.g. dermatofibrosarcoma, Kaposi's sarcoma, epithelioid sarcoma). **Or malignant transformation of chronic wounds** (usually to squamous cell carcinoma).

**You must think outside of the box!**

> **"Try to fit each wound you see into one of the common groups but don't forget that many are of mixed etiology."**

# Chapter 3

## Wound healing and non-healing — why are these wounds 'problematic'?

*The wound is a window into the body.*

**Now, when you know what wound bearers have been dumped in the 'cesspool', before fishing them out and attending to their wounds, let us dwell briefly on the mechanisms of wound healing and what factors could interfere with your therapeutic efforts.**

### Mechanisms of wound healing

**As promised, I will limit myself to essential basics.** The physiological process of wound healing occurs in four key overlapping phases, which are described in ■ Table 3.1.

#### Epidermal advancement

**This is a crucial step in the proliferative phase, during which epidermal cells (keratinocytes) epithelialize the wound surface, restoring the skin's barrier function.** These cells migrate primarily from the wound edges. Still, intact hair follicles and sweat glands may contribute to the epithelization, thus the tiny islands of 'new skin' you will see occasionally at the center of a granulating wound (typically in second-degree burns). **Your main job is to allow unhindered progress of epidermal advancement.**

**Table 3.1. The physiological phases of wound healing.**

| Phase | Goal | Process |
|---|---|---|
| **1. Hemostasis (immediate)** | Arrest bleeding and initiate repair | • Vasoconstriction<br>• Platelets form a clot<br>• Clotting factors produce a fibrin mesh |
| **2. Inflammatory (hours to days)** | Remove debris and bacteria | • Neutrophils and macrophages arrive to clean and phagocytose non-viable tissue and microorganisms<br>• Wound is inflamed and painful |
| **3. Proliferative (days to weeks)** | Repair the wound | • Fibroblasts produce collagen and extracellular matrix<br>• Angiogenesis to produce capillaries<br>• Keratinocytes restore the surface<br>• The wound starts to granulate and heal |
| **4. Maturing/remodeling (weeks to months)** | Produce a strong scar | • Further build-up of collagen.<br>• Wound is contracting and healing |

**What is the pace of epithelial advancement?**

- **Under optimal conditions (e.g. a 'clean' laceration in a healthy patient and healthy tissues)**, the keratinocytes migrate across the wound bed at a rate of 0.5-1mm per day. Thus, a superficial, half-centimeter wound may heal within 7-10 days.
- **Chronic wounds (defined by some as wounds that do not heal within 4-12 weeks — typically those referred to your wound care clinic) do not heal as well**. Here, epithelial advancement is usually stalled due to the many factors discussed below. The rate of healing varies depending on the specific characteristics of the wound, the patient, and the quality of your wound management. **In general, only half of chronic wounds heal within 3-4 months. Some take longer, and some never heal.**
- An example: a healing rate of 0.5mm per week of a venous ulcer suggests that your treatment is successful!

## Factors which prevent the healing of wounds

**Numerous factors (■ Table 3.2) play a role, usually in combination, to impede the physiological process of wound healing — interfering in one or more of the key stages stated above — thus rendering the wound 'chronic'.**

**Table 3.2. Factors which prevent the healing of wounds.**

| The patient | The wound | External/iatrogenic factors |
|---|---|---|
| • Advanced age<br>• Obesity<br>• Diabetes<br>• Smoking<br>• Immunosuppressive state (HIV, cancer...)<br>• Malnutrition | • Ischemia<br>• Devitalized tissue/products<br>• Obstacles to epidermal migration<br>• Infection/contamination<br>• Local edema<br>• Excessive dryness or moisture<br>• Repeated or constant trauma/pressure<br>• Foreign body<br>• Fistula | • Drugs (steroids, chemotherapy, anticoagulants...)<br>• Radiation<br>• Poor care<br>• Non-compliance<br>• Social-economic deprivation |

### Patient-related factors

There is no need to dwell on the 'basics' such as that **older patients** experience slower healing due to diminished cell proliferation and vascularization; that **systemic disease like diabetes** impairs tissue perfusion, the immune response to infection and epithelial migration; that **immunosuppression** by disease and drugs delays inflammation and reduces the ability to fight infection; that **obesity** increases inflammation, reduces tissue perfusion and places mechanical stress on the tissues; and that **smoking** decreases blood flow and oxygen delivery to the wound. That **malnutrition** slows/prevents wound healing is yet another 'basic' but is not always 'obvious'. I remember a young college kid, healthy, well-fed, and athletic, with an open sacral wound following pilonidal surgery, which 'refused' to heal despite all our efforts. We then realized that the guy sustained himself solely by devouring hamburgers and fries or cheese/ham sandwiches. "I don't like veggies and fruits," he declared. **He lacked the vitamins essential for wound healing!**

## Wound-related factors

The following are the local wound factors that prevent the wound from healing. **I will describe each of the items separately, but do understand that, in most cases, such factors coexist, promoting each other while simultaneously frustrating your healing efforts.**

### *Ischemia*

**Tissue ischemia is the 'A' of the 'ABC' of wound healing. When the blood supply and $O_2$ delivery to the wound are reduced — forget about being able to heal anything.** Ischemia can be obvious: think about the clearly ischemic below-knee necrotic amputation stump after failed attempts at limb revascularization. **But often ischemia is inconspicuous or 'relative'**: think about a pressure sore on the heel of a diabetic patient — the foot appears well perfused, there is enough perfusion to keep the foot alive, but not enough to heal the wound.

### *Devitalized tissue/products*

**Necrotic tissue** (skin, subcutaneous fat, muscle) residing within the wound prevents the healing process from progressing. The same is true for **residual blood clots** and their products. **Without thorough debridement, the wound won't heal, stalling in an 'obstinate' inflammatory state — infection sets in, and the vicious circle will continue.**

### *Obstacles to epidermal migration*

**The wound won't heal if its edges do not permit migration of epithelial cells from the periphery of the wound.** Rolled-elevated edges (*epibole*), a surrounding callous, hypergranulating and/or undermined tunneling edges — all prevent migration and must be addressed.

### *Infection/contamination*

**Infection with various microorganisms sets chaos at each of the stages of the wound healing process; chaotic as well is how the literature covers this topic; even more chaos exists in how contamination or infection of such wounds is dealt with in clinical practice** (did you see any patient referred to the wound care clinic who did not receive already a course or two, or more, of some oral antibiotics?). Here and in ➲ Chapters 5-7, I will try to impose some order on that chaos:

- **Most, if not all, open wounds are contaminated with bacteria. Period. If you swab a persistent open wound for culture, it will grow some bacteria. But it doesn't mean that the wound is infected!**
- **Any chronic open wound represents a 'microbial continuum'.**

- **Contamination**: bacteria 'sleep' in the wound, but they are not active.
- **Colonization**: the bacteria 'wake up' and replicate, which may impair healing.
- **Critical colonization**: a 'load' of bacteria impairs wound healing.
- **Infection**: bacteria invade tissue, with local (and systemic) features of infection present.

**In theory, this 'continuum' appears appealing. Still, in practice, 'infection' is obvious, but the distinction between the first three entities is less clear, cumbersome, and often calls for an 'empirical' approach.**

**The problem of a biofilm**: the biofilm is a layer of microorganisms encased in a self-produced matrix, adhering to the bed of a non-healing wound, **shielding bacteria from local immune mechanisms and antibiotics, and sustaining low-grade inflammation that, in turn, stalls wound healing.** Biofilms are described as a shiny, gelatinous 'film' forming on the wound bed, but in practice, **you do not 'see' a biofilm — you suspect it! Even when eradicated, biofilms recur rapidly — within 24 hours.**

**Infection may set in in deeper structures — below the wound**; for example, osteomyelitis below a toe ulcer in a diabetic patient, or infection of a mesh below a wound that fails to heal after umbilical hernia repair. **If you do not deal with the infected bone, if you do not remove the infected mesh — the wounds will never heal!**

### *Local edema*

**Edema is a constant enemy of wound healing.** In some instances, the swelling/congestion of the tissues plays a significant role in the genesis of the wound (e.g. venous stasis ulcer, the 'big boy' syndrome, etc.); in some situations, it is a byproduct of the problem (e.g. post-traumatic wounds); in many others it represents a chronic underlying problem (e.g. congestive heart failure, the paraplegic wheelchair-ridden patient).

**Edema impairs oxygen and nutrient delivery**, delays cellular activity, prevents evacuation of byproducts of tissue destruction and inflammation, provides a breeding environment for bacteria, and promotes maceration and breakdown of surrounding skin. **It produces leaking wounds that are difficult to manage.**

> **Remember: swollen, edematous tissues do not heal. To achieve healing, you must reduce the swelling by whatever measures are available.**

### *Dryness or excessive moisture*

You will see many patients arriving at your wound care clinic with an exposed wound, covered with a dry scab. "My doctor said to leave the wound open to fresh air... let the scab fall off..." they would say. **But this is wrong! Dry wounds impair cell migration, thereby delaying epithelization.**

**Conversely, moist wounds promote 'autolytic debridement' (e.g. the evacuation of non-viable tissue by immune cells), preserve growth factors, support angiogenesis and collagen production, while minimizing pain. However, excessive moisture is harmful — the same harms described above concerning 'tissue edema'.**

> **Remember: moisture control is crucial. Avoid 'dryness' and 'wetness' — find the right balance to keep the wound 'just moist' — to be discussed in ➲ Chapter 7.**

### *Repeated or constant trauma/pressure*

**This is obvious**: the heel ulcer won't heal if the shoe continues rubbing on it. The sacral decubitus will progress if the patient continues sitting in his wheelchair in the same position all day.

### *Foreign body*

This is a no-brainer as well: the groin wound will persist as long as the infected vascular graft remains exposed at the bottom of the wound. The wound you have been managing now for a month with a 'wound VAC' won't heal until you fish out the tiny piece of 'black sponge' the visiting home nurse has left in it inadvertently.

*Fistula*

Wounds that are constantly draining the corrosive fluids of fistulas (e.g. gastrointestinal, pancreatic, salivary fistulas) will never heal until the fistula dries up.

**All such wound-related factors end in dysregulated healing mechanisms: instead of transitioning to the proliferative phase, the wound remains stuck in an inflammatory state.**

## External and iatrogenic factors

External factors that may have a negative impact on wound healing become clear to you after taking the basic history:

- **Drugs**: certain drugs inhibit wound healing through various mechanisms. **Immunosuppressants** (used to prevent transplant organ rejection or autoimmune diseases) can impair the inflammatory response. **Corticosteroids** reduce inflammation and slow down wound contraction and collagen production. That **non-steroidal anti-inflammatory drugs (NSAIDs)** are anti-inflammatory is obvious. Some **chemotherapy drugs** (used to treat cancer) interfere with cell proliferation, collagen synthesis, and the immune response. **Anti-rheumatoid drugs** (e.g. colchicine, methotrexate, and even aspirin) slow tissue repair through their anti-inflammatory actions. **And did you know that anticoagulants also slow wound healing? They do so by interfering with the early 'hemostasis phase' of wound healing, which requires the production of a clot and a fibrin mesh**. That such drugs can limit and complicate wound debridement is obvious. It is significant because most patients presenting to the wound care clinic are already receiving some form of anticoagulation (indicated or not).
- **Radiation**: previously irradiated tissue is poorly vascularized and fibrotic. It is prone to injury and poor healing.
- **Poor care**: I see examples of inappropriate or misguided wound care almost daily: insufficient debridement, overzealous packing, incorrect use of wound VACs, bizarre dressings, omission of compression devices, and neglect of patient-related and 'external/iatrogenic' factors — the list is long.
- **Non-compliance**: this is common as well. A typical example — patients are reluctant to wear compression stockings. **Remember: swollen tissues don't heal**.
- **Social-economic deprivation**: unfortunately, chronic wounds tend to develop in 'underprivileged' populations, lacking family support and access to healthcare, or unable to navigate the system.

All these factors, if not appropriately assessed (➲ Chapter 4) and not treated optimally (see ➲ Parts II and III), will disrupt the fine-tuned biological process of healing, stalling it or preventing it indefinitely.

> **"The key principle is: the wound needs oxygen to heal. Anything that prevents oxygen delivery to the wound (e.g. poor blood supply, edema, necrotic tissue, old blood, bacteria) impedes healing. Our job is to optimize oxygen delivery to the wound and 'fine-tune' the process of healing. All the rest is secondary."**

# Chapter 4

## Assessment of the patients and their wounds

*Wounds cannot be cured without searching.*

**Francis Bacon, 1561-1626**

Typically, many 'problem wounds' tend to 'fall between the cracks' until they finally land at your wound care clinic. Let us now see how to assess them, and to decide how to proceed with their treatment.

**You can proceed in an organized fashion, which allows you (within 30-60 minutes) to answer the following questions.**

- **What type of wound is it** (■ Table 2.1)?
- **Which of the factors that prevent healing are present** (■ Table 3.2)?
- **Would the wound be healable in your hands?** Or do you need to refer the patient immediately (e.g. for radical surgical debridement, revascularization procedure, or amputation)?
- **Would your role be limited only to 'maintenance' of the wound or 'palliative' treatment** (e.g. ischemic ulcer with no revascularization option, decubitus ulcer in a terminal cancer patient)?

## The patient and their wound history

**History-taking is crucial for capturing all patient-related and external factors that prevent healing, as listed in ■ Table 3.2.** Much of it can be done before the encounter with the patient by reviewing his electronic medical record (EMR). It is often easier said than done, given the typically crowded EMR. However, I make a special effort to review all recent encounters with the referring physicians: previous notes from any wound care clinic, if available; all recent lab work (e.g. blood count, albumin levels, HbA1c); and relevant ancillary tests (e.g. Ankle-Brachial Index [ABI]) and imaging (e.g. X-rays, MRIs, CT angiography or MRIs of the foot in the case of a foot ulcer).

Unfortunately, some important information may be buried deep under the loads of crap included in the EMR. Some of those patients' records are longer than the Bible, and some patients are referred from 'elsewhere' with incomplete records. **If you don't dig deeply, you will miss things.** Below is an example from my own experience.

**A female presented with an ischemic and heavily infected stump of an above-knee amputation.** I could see the end of the femur sticking out at the stump (■ Figure 4.1). Typically, her records showed numerous previous procedures attempting to 'save' her limb — vascular bypasses, stent placements, staged amputations (toes, foot, below knee, above knee). The EMR contained an endless list of imaging procedures and their interpretations, which I scrolled through. **I decided to remove the ischemic stump and took her for a high-thigh amputation.** I fashioned well-vascularized flaps and started sawing the femur. Still, the electric saw refused to cut through — a horrible surprise! The intraoperative image provided the explanation (■ Figure 4.2); it is impossible to cut through a titanium rod! I completed the amputation of the flaps (■ Figure 4.3) and shipped the patient to an orthopedic center, where the rod was removed and the amputation revised. **A traumatic event for the patient, embarrassing to the surgeon. The fact that the EMR is a mile long is not an excuse!**

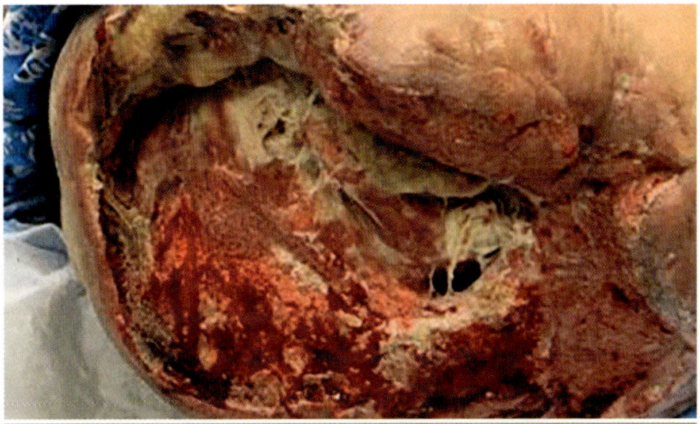

Figure 4.1. Infected, necrotic above-knee amputation stump, with the tip of the femur sticking out.

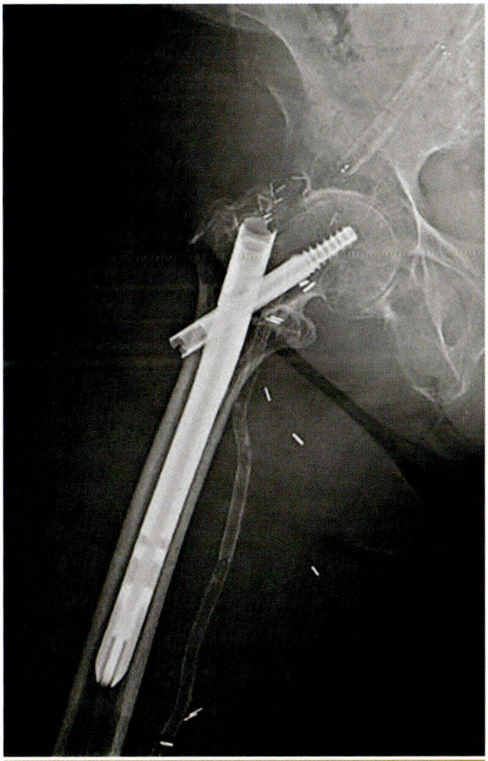

Figure 4.2. Intraoperative image showing the titanium rod within the femur.

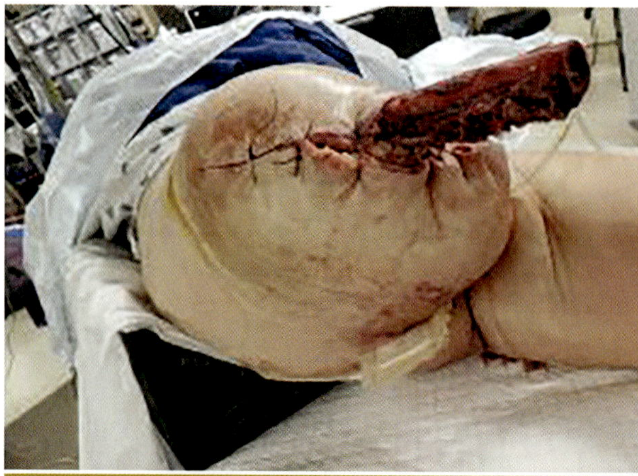

Figure 4.3. High-thigh amputation 'completed'.

## The wound

**Next you will assess the wound(s).**

I often see in charts from other 'wound care providers' a lengthy description of each wound they encounter, in the form of elaborate check lists and/or excessively descriptive text. I find it unnecessary, and I keep it simple. All you must note, during each encounter, is the following:

- **Location of the wound(s).** Where exactly is it situated?
- **Size.** Measured in centimeters: length X, width X, depth X. Length refers to the vertical axis of the body and limb, the width to the transverse axis. To measure the depth, use a sterile cotton tip or instrument.
- **Edges of the wound. Are they non-viable, surrounded by callous, rolling/folding inwards (*epibole*) or undermined, or tunneling — all factors preventing epidermal advancement?** Undermining is measured with a sterile cotton tip, its location referring to the clock. For example: "wound edges are undermined for 2cm at 11 to 2 o'clock".
- **Base of the wound. What do you see at the base of the wound? What is the condition of the tissue?** Is it healthy-pink, covered with granulation tissue? Is it covered with yellow or brown necrotic slough? Is it frankly necrotic-black? Can you observe any deep structures exposed — bone, tendones, arterial graft, intestine (**bad news!**)?

- **What does the wound produce?** Is the wound dry or wet? (The patient may have already complained that his dressings are constantly wet and dripping…) **What type of exudate do you see: serous, serosanguinous, purulent? The 'wetness' (moisture) of the wound is best estimated by looking at the discarded dressings — don't let your assistant dump it before you can see it!** Look at the color of the exudate — greenish discoloration suggests infection with *Pseudomonas*. And yes — **do smell the wound and dressing**.
- **What is the condition/integrity of the surrounding skin (the periwound)?** Rarely in these patients is the skin in the vicinity of the wound entirely 'normal'. Look for surrounding **erythema** (cellulitis), **bruising** (injury, hematoma), **stasis dermatitis** (venous ulcer), **maceration** (inside folds of skin in the morbidly obese), and **edema**. **Are there any varicose veins present** suggesting a varicose/stasis ulcer? (To see the varicosities let the patient stand up.) Get an impression of the **patient's general hygiene**, which would reflect on their ability to self-care for their wound.

## Assessment of perfusion

This is crucial because, as I mentioned above, at least two-thirds of the wounds seen at the wound care clinic involve the lower extremities. So, you not only have to think like a podiatrist, but also like a vascular surgeon.

**What really matters is the examination of peripheral pulses. I start with checking the foot pulses (dorsalis pedis and tibialis posterior). If intensely palpable, I know that the perfusion of the feet is satisfactory. Period. No further ancillary testing is needed**.

**If I don't feel the pulses**, which is often tricky in grossly edematous limbs, I listen to them with a **handheld Doppler**. Loud arterial signals are reassuring. However, audible arterial signals do not provide quantitative information about the adequacy of perfusion — is it sufficient to support healing of the wound? **Therefore, if the pulses are not palpable and I suspect an 'element of ischemia', I refer the patient for a 'formal' ABI (Ankle-Brachial Index) study, which objectively assesses ankle and toe pressure**. Based on the ABI study and the clinical situation, I may proceed with **CT angiography** including images of the peripheral run-off. (See ➲ Chapter 15 on ischemic ulcers.)

**Be aware that the ABI may be unreliable in diabetic patients in whom the peripheral arteries are calcified and non-compressible, giving falsely**

**high readings. Also, palpable peripheral pulses do not entirely exclude ischemia in these patients. The Toe-Brachial Index is more reliable because the toe arteries are rarely calcified** (➲ Chapter 15).

Some would advocate other 'perfusion tests' to measure the quality of perfusion to the skin (e.g. transcutaneous oxygen measurement, laser Doppler flowmetry), but, as always, the number of tests ordered does not equate to a better quality of care and outcomes.

**Recognize the term 'relative ischemia': arterial perfusion is sufficient to maintain viability and function of an intact limb but not to support healing.**

## Assessment of sensation

**Individuals with diminished sensation in their legs and feet due to peripheral neuropathy are prone to chronic wounds**. They don't feel when the new shoes rub their toes, or when the wood stove is too close to their feet. The leading cause for neuropathy in the patients you encounter is diabetes; other, less common causes are neural spine injuries, alcoholism, chemotherapy — the list is long.

Most patients may have been referred with an already known diagnosis of peripheral neuropathy with symptoms of numbness, tingling, and burning pain in their feet. You can confirm the diagnosis by examination: **light touch** (with a cotton wisp or a monofilament thread), **pain perception** (with a pin), **temperature sensation** (with any cold/hot item), **vibration sensation** (with a tuning fork placed on a bony prominence) and **position sensation** (does the patient feel whether the toe is pointing up or down?).

About the 'motor' consequences of neuropathy to the affected limb — what it does to the structure of the foot — contributing to the formation of ulcers, go to ➲ Chapter 14 on the 'diabetic foot'.

## Assessment of infection

**It's not a big deal to diagnose an infection in an acute surgical or traumatic wound (pain, pus, redness, swelling surrounding cellulitis). But recognizing infection in a chronic wound is not as simple — it is prone to uncertainties, delays, confusion, and therapeutic chaos.**

I mentioned previously (➲ Chapter 3) the 'microbial continuum' in chronic wounds, where '**contamination**' (remember, all chronic open wounds are 'contaminated'!) is clinically meaningless, but that a certain degree of '**colonization**' can delay wound healing. **The big problem is how to distinguish between these entities — at what point does 'contamination' becomes 'colonization' and 'colonization' represent 'latent' or 'low-grade' infection, which can impact wound healing. How do we decide whether to treat it and by what method**?

## Obvious infection

**The presence of exudate (and its color — greenish, suggesting the presence of *Pseudomonas*), erythema, and debris point to superficial infection of the wound**. Add to it local signs (e.g. tenderness, cellulitis, malodor) and systemic signs. Add to it lab findings (e.g. temperature, leukocytosis, elevated CRP, etc.) and imaging (suggesting underlying osteomyelitis), and you know that you are dealing with a 'deeper' infection. **In such a situation, there is no question how to proceed**: you must drain and debride the wound, take a culture and start antibiotics, either orally or intravenously, depending on the extent of the infection (see ➲ Chapter 6).

## Non-obvious (latent/low-grade) infection

**You suspect it because the wound is not healing — it is stuck in the 'inflammatory phase'**. There are no apparent signs of infection (keep in mind that clinical signs of infection can be subtle or absent in immunosuppressed or diabetic patients who cannot mount an inflammatory response, and remember the 'non-visible' biofilm), but you don't observe any activity in the wound — no granulation tissue, no epidermal advancement across it. You don't know whether the wound is 'significantly colonized' by bacteria, 'infected', or just 'contaminated'.

## How to proceed?

- **When you diagnose deep/spreading infection** you must admit the patient, start i.v. antibiotics, and call the surgeon (that is if you are not a surgeon) so he can plan surgical debridement.
- **If you observe an obvious 'local' infection** you must start oral antibiotics and drain the wound.
- **Which 'empirical antibiotics' should be given** will be discussed in ➲ Chapter 6.

**These decisions are 'easy' but what to do when you suspect infection but there are no signs? The next step is to take a culture from the wound.**

## Qualitative versus quantitative wound culture

What are the differences between 'qualitative' and 'quantitative' wound cultures?

- **A quantitative wound culture** requires submission of a tissue biopsy or aspirated fluid to the lab, where it undergoes extensive processing techniques. Results are typically reported as colony-forming units (CFU) per gram of tissue or milliliter of fluid. **This way it can distinguish between colonization and infection — high counts (>$10^5$ CFU/g of tissue) suggest infection.**
- **A qualitative wound culture** is typically swab-based. It only identifies the presence and type of microorganisms; **it won't imply whether the wound is infected or 'only' colonized.**
- **Semiquantitative wound culture techniques** use methods which report the 'density' of bacteria in the specimen as 'trace', 'few', 'moderate' or 'abundant'.

Although the **quantitative** methods are considered the 'gold standard', the less invasive, easier, and cost-effective **qualitative methods are predominantly used in clinical practice**. Some labs offer **semiquantitative** data as well; for example, the reports I receive from our lab may describe, in addition to the specific organism cultured and its susceptibility to a list of antibiotics, terms like "light growth of *Staphylococcus aureus*" or "moderate mixed skin flora" (See ➲ Chapter 6 for details).

## How to obtain a wound culture

**The technique of swabbing the wounds for culture is often performed incorrectly**: people simply dip the swab into the wound and *voilà* — "we found bacteria, infection, let's treat it!"

**The 'correct' technique you should use has been described by Norman S. Levine. It is more reflective of the actual tissue bacterial burden than simply 'poking' or 'swabbing' the surface of the wound. Here is how you do it:**

- **Avoid taking specimens from exudate, necrotic material or eschar — they will always be positive!** Thus, take a culture only after you have debrided the wound.

- Clean the wound with saline.
- Rotate the swab over a 1 $cm^2$ area at the base of the wound, applying pressure to express fluid.
- Don't let the swab touch the periphery of the wounds and your gloves.

So now, after submitting the culture, you must wait for the results. Meanwhile, you must use your clinical judgment to decide whether to 'treat' the suspected infection or 'critical colonization'. And even when the results of culture become available you may not get a 'definitive' answer. **Now you understand that modern wound care is as much an art as science**. Many decisions taken are empirical!

On how to interpret and act upon the results of wound culture, see ➲ Chapter 6.

## Assessment of functional, psychosocial, and system factors

**There are numerous other factors, in addition to those detailed hitherto, that directly impact the healing of a wound**. You won't be able to discover and attempt to correct all of them during the first encounter, but sooner or later, you will have to do so; otherwise, the wound won't not only improve but can even deteriorate. Many questions must be asked and answered:

- **Mobility**: is the patient mobile or sedentary? It will affect the type of leg compression to use. Can the 'big boy' reach down and wash his feet? Or does he need help?
- **Pressure injury risk**: is the patient wheelchair-ridden? What type of wheelchair? Are precautions taken to avoid pressure wounds on the buttocks? How does he sleep? Are the heels protected to prevent pressure injury?
- **Cognitive capacity and mood**: does the patient comprehend his situation and take an active role in his treatment? Is he depressed or apathetic? Should it be addressed?
- **Compliance**: does the patient and/or his family follow your instructions?
- **Social-economic deprivation: like with health care in general, patients belonging to low socio-economic strata are much more prone to chronic wounds and associated comorbidities**. What is

the patient's living conditions? Does he have running water? Is the heating/cooling adequate? Who will transport him to your wound care clinic? Does he live alone? Are there any friends nearby who can help dress his back wound? Are there any children who can assist?

- **Access to care**: what type of medical insurance does the patient have, if any? If not, would he be able to pay for even the cheapest antibiotic agent you prescribe? Can he afford the 'copay' required for each visit? How much? Should you see him less frequently? Can he pay for any of the 'fancy dressings' or should you try something 'simpler/cheaper'?
- **Quality of care**: does the staff of the nursing home follow your wound care instructions? Or does the patient develop additional pressure sores during follow-up? Are the 'home care providers' up to the job? Or do they continue packing the wound too tightly so it will never heal?

## Is the wound malignant?

**Skin cancers may present as, or be confused for, a 'chronic wound'. Conversely, skin cancers may develop in a chronic wound. Both situations are rare, but if missed, can lead to advanced local lesions, complicating treatments and increasing morbidity**. Experienced clinicians are unlikely to confuse skin cancers with chronic wounds because most skin cancers have a characteristic appearance. And anyway, they know that any spontaneous wounds (appearing without apparent cause) should be removed or biopsied, immediately or when they fail to heal rapidly. **On the other hand, even seasoned specialists occasionally do not recognize cancers developing in chronic wounds**.

Skin cancer (usually a squamous cell carcinoma) developing in a chronic wound is referred to as a '**Marjolin's ulcer**'. Typically, the malignant transformation occurs in wounds (e.g. venous/stasis ulcers or fistula-in-ano) that have been present for years. However, cases of 'acute' malignant transformation already after a year have been described. Exophytic growth, bleeding, and excessive granulation tissue extending beyond the margins are suggestive findings. **You should think about it in any longstanding wound that should heal but doesn't. A punch biopsy is diagnostic**.

## Documentation

**Adequate documentation of your assessment of the patient and their wound, your treatment of it, and your plans is crucial.** It is essential not only to satisfy the **regulatory requirements** of your employers and to **get paid** for what you do (oh, yes, the 'fee for service' or payment based on 'productivity' is a horrible system), **but it's mainly to help you provide optimal and continued care for the wound. For when you treat 20 leg ulcers per week — each massive or indurated limb looking the same — only carefully recorded information would remind you of the details of the patient seen yet again, to monitor his progress, to change course, and to avoid repeating unnecessary tests.** In addition, detailed documentation helps your partner (or competitor, or other specialists) to take over care of the patient, if necessary. **Undoubtedly, in chronic wound care, with its diagnostic uncertainty and treatment complexity, documentation is the basis for continuity of care and responsibility.**

## What should represent 'adequate documentation'?

The way clinicians document what they do differs from place to place, depending on local 'culture'. In specific environments, particularly where EMRs are not used, and people must still invest energy to move their hands on paper, one still may see laconic documentation such as: "A 55-year-old obese diabetic patient with a 1cm recurrent varicose ulcer on the right medial malleolus. Good peripheral pulses. Wound cleaned. Unna boot re-applied. See next week."

Frankly, there is nothing wrong with such brief, narrative-based documentation. The wound will heal regardless of whether the documentation is a single paragraph or includes a well-structured 1000 words (often a copy and paste) in an EMR-based encounter note. **However, in our current environment, much more is mandatory.** It is required by credentialing bodies (your charting is being monitored and audited by 'big brother'), Medicare, and other payors (e.g. the wound VAC that you order won't be 'approved' if detailed information of the wound is not listed). **The question is how much more?**

- **The answer is to avoid over-documentation.** Often, I see patients' notes from other wound care providers, which require endless scrolling to find relevant information.

- **By necessity, the information documented after your first encounter tends to be longer.** But avoid copying and pasting whole segments into each of your follow-up notes (as some people do) to serve as a 'reminder' or to show how 'thorough' you are. You have documented adequate perfusion of the feet during the first encounter, and the ABI study was normal — there is no need to repeat it.
- **Be practical and record only clinically relevant information.** Don't repeat yourself and tell long stories. There is no need to mention after each time you scrape the wound with a scalpel (e.g. 'selective debridement'), that "hemostasis was obtained with pressure" and that "the patient tolerated the debridement well" — even if you can easily insert a 'macro' containing such and other useless phrases.
- **Remember: no one, not even you, will read again all that you have documented.** Besides, you don't want to spend more than 5 minutes on documentation when the typical encounter lasts 30 minutes.

**Here is how I document the 'wound encounter'** (you can create a 'macro' to include the listed 'items':

- **General statement summarizing the factors which impacts on wound healing.** For example: "This is an 85-year-old man, diabetic, morbidly obese, wheelchair-ridden, peripheral arterial disease, metastatic lung cancer stage 4, on warfarin."
- **Timeline.** For example: "The wound developed 3 months ago. Under my treatment for 6 weeks. Last seen a week ago."
- **Etiology.** For example: "Venous ulcer", "pressure ulcer", "mixed etiology".
- **Wound assessment**:
  - **wound number**: if there are a few wounds, then each requires separate documentation — "wound 1", "wound 2", and so on;
  - **wound location**;
  - **wound length X, width X, depth X** (in cm);
  - **wound undermining** (location of undermining in cm — e.g. "2-9 o'clock");
  - **tunneling** (in cm: how long, from where to where);
  - **level of tissue damage: "partial-thickness"** (involving epidermis and dermis only) versus **"full-thickness"**, when the subcutaneous fat is exposed. Staging the level of a specific type of ulcer (pressure, venous, diabetic) is discussed in Part III;
  - **wound tissue**: the type of tissue at the base of the wound (granulation, necrotic, slough, eschar, fibrin);

  - **wound drainage/moisture**: is the wound dry? Or is it productive/wet? With what? Serous fluid, pus, blood? How much?
  - **wound margins**: regular, necrotic, elevated (*epibole*)?
  - **peri-wound skin**: intact, erythema, maceration, induration, callus formation.
- **Infection**: local or systemic signs, lab values, culture results.
- **Goal of healing**: based on your assessment hitherto, and the progress of the wound, you can now classify it in the following categories:
  - **healable wounds**: blood supply adequate; underlying etiologies (e.g. venous hypertension, edema) controlled; no major local or systemic barriers to healing;
  - **maintenance wounds**: the wound is potentially healable but there are significant barriers preventing progress (e.g. patient non-compliant, refusing to wear compression stockings or skips appointments);
  - **non-healable wounds** (e.g. a terminal cancer patient with bedsores, a 500-pound wheelchair-bound patient with sacral decubitus who 'eats himself to death'). Here, your goal will be 'palliation' — see ➲ Chapter 10.
- **Wound care: how did you treat the wound during the encounter?**
  - irrigated with?
  - applied local treatment (ointments, creams)?
  - dressed ('moisture control') with?
  - covered ('secondary dressing') with?
  - wrapped with?
  - compression with?
- **Debridement: what type (e.g. selective, non-selective, see ➲ Chapter 5)?** Some people prefer to describe any debridement using instruments under a separate heading of 'procedure note'.
- **The cliché, "a picture is worth a thousand words" is especially relevant in wound care. The truth is that a carefully captured image of the wound, before and after debridement, could replace exhaustive description of the wound and its progress over time. I use it obsessively (■ Figure 4.4).**
- **Summary and plan**: are you 'happy' with the healing process or is the wound 'stalled'? Do you need to change course? What are the next steps — antibiotics, images, ordering wound VAC, discussion with 'home care' or a nursing home, referrals to another subspeciality? **And when do you want to see the patient again?**

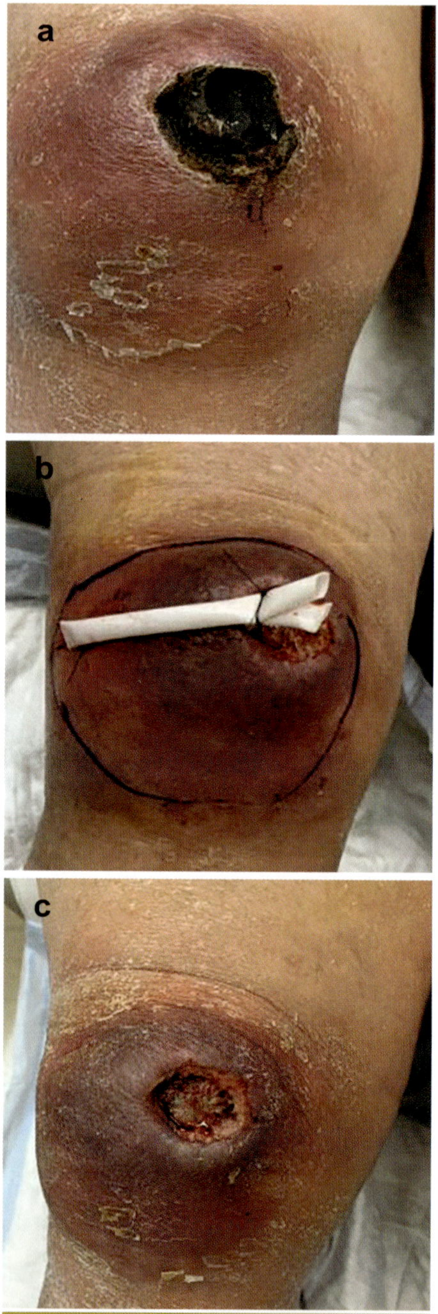


**Figure 4.4. Images showing progression of a wound caused by a post-traumatic knee hematoma over 3 weeks. a) Before evacuation of the knee hematoma. b) After evacuation. c) After 2 weeks of wound VAC treatment.**

## Wound healing 'scoring systems'

The literature recommends various 'scoring systems' to assess the healing progress of multiple types of wounds. What is true of many other scoring systems developed in different clinical disciplines is also true in wound care — they are cumbersome, and clinicians do not adopt them. Nor do I.

**I spent more than 1000 words here on how to document wound care. In most cases, an encounter note of approximately 250 words would suffice.**

> **"Documentation should support patient care, not just billing requirements — less is more, and short is sweet."**

# PART II

# General concepts of wound management

*Wound care is like cooking.*

While the principles of wound care are well established, the actual care is subjected to numerous dogmas and personal preferences, many based on rudimentary and conflicting evidence. **Therefore, you should provide wound care as if you were a private chef cooking a gourmet dinner for an opulent client.** The master chef selects the dishes and ingredients to suit the customer's decadent palate. Similarly, you must adjust your course of action, and the materials used to the individual patient and the circumstances of their wound. **The basics of wound care are universal, but each wound needs specific consideration. If the soup turns too spicy or the steak is overdone, the chef will discard the product and try again. It's the same in wound care: if, after a week or two, the wound is not showing signs of improvement, you must reevaluate and try something else.**

Here, in Part II, we will discuss the general concepts of management of ALL types of wounds. In Part III we will dwell on the management of specific sorts of wounds.

Generally, I dislike acronyms, there are too many of them and they don't add much to what we do, except perhaps helping people studying for exams. **But TIME is a useful, 'cute' acronym because it encompasses the basics of wound care.**

- **T**: refers to **TISSUE** management, which means debridement.
- **I**: refers to **INFECTION** — all we have to do to prevent bacteria interfering with healing.
- **M**: refers to **MOISTURE** — this includes keeping the wound moist to allow epithelization, removing excessive exudate which delays repair mechanisms, but preventing dryness/desiccation or excessive wetness/edema that also hinders healing. **Optimal moisture balance is crucial.**
- **E**: refers to **epithelial** edge advancement. Epithelial cells should be able to migrate from the surrounding skin to cover the wound bed. Thus, wound edges that obstruct such migration must be dealt with.

**Now, let us discuss how to achieve the TIME components.**

# Chapter 5

## Wound debridement

*The act of 'debridement' — the removal of necrotic non-viable tissue, and/or 'freshening' the wound is a keystone of management.*

Let's start with the T of TIME.

**What does debridement achieve?** It exposes the wound bed for accurate assessment (e.g. how deep is the wound and what structures lie at its bed?); it eradicates non-viable tissue and exudate; it reduces bacterial load and removes the biofilm; it stimulates wound edge activity and cellular migration; it improves the effectiveness of topical agents and dressings — **all together it restores a healthy wound bed, eliminating local barriers to the healing process**.

### Nomenclature

**The literature describes numerous methods of 'debridement'**: 'sharp', 'surgical', 'selective', 'non-selective', 'biological', 'enzymatic', 'chemical', 'autolytic', 'mechanical', 'conservative', etc.

**But please do not allow yourself to be confused by all of these and be practical: there is only one *real* method of wound debridement, and it is surgical** (non-surgeons can call it 'sharp', that is if the term 'surgical' sounds too pretentious). **It is either surgical 'selective', or 'non-selective'. The term 'surgical' means that you are using instruments (scalpel, forceps, curette...).**

You may wonder why I am somehow 'dismissive' of the other methods. Let's see:

- **Biological debridement** refers to the use of live **maggots** to gobble up the necrotic tissue and exudate. My late father was a surgeon in the Russian Army during World War II. He used to recount the wounded soldiers arriving at his field hospital after many days of journey from the front in 'hospital trains'. The wounds in those who survived the ordeal swarmed with fat maggots under the filthy dressings and casts, but were pink and clean. The maggots did a great job! But procuring maggots from the single laboratory that offers them in the USA, maintaining them alive, and applying them to wounds is complex and costly — not practical for the average wound care clinic. Unless, however, the maggots are already 'supplied' by the patient (■ Figure 5.1).

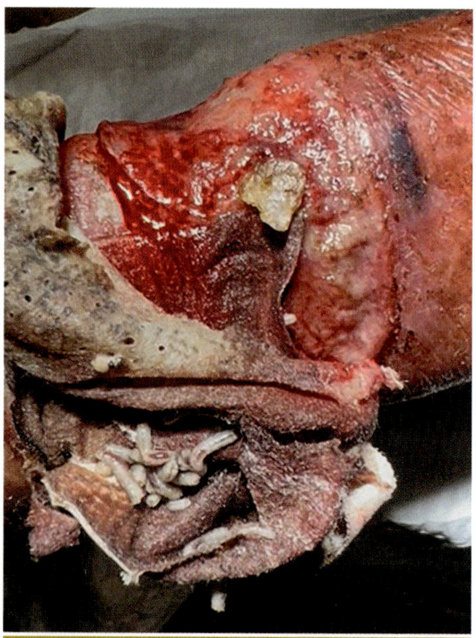

**Figure 5.1. Maggots on a neglected forearm wound. The patient presented 2 weeks after injury with a 'self-treated' wound. Note how clean the wound is under the filthy dressing!**

- **Enzymatic debridement** refers to the use of a collagenase-containing **ointment**. Only one such product is FDA-approved in the USA. It allegedly dissolves the collagen in necrotic tissue, without interfering with healthy/healing tissues. A prospective randomized study conducted in patients with diabetic ulcers, comparing the use of this agent against one of the 'silver dressings', claimed that after 6 weeks of treatment, the 'ointment group' had a 62% reduction in the size of the ulcer as opposed to a 40% reduction in the 'silver dressing' group. Each study group consisted of 51 patients, gathered from 14 sites! **I mention these details only to show you (again) how poor the quality of evidence supporting most of the 'novel products' advocated for wound care is.** The cost of the ointment for 1 month of use would be a few hundred US dollars. Most insurance companies are reluctant to cover it. **A scalpel is cheaper and faster.**

- **Mechanical debridement** refers to a few methods that use force to separate or break necrotic tissue without the use of instruments. **Irrigating** the wound under some pressure and *gently* **scrubbing** it with a piece of gauze (I use moist 4 x 4 gauze) should be part of your routine wound care anyway. **Low-frequency ultrasound** has been recommended for wound debridement. But, again, any evidence of its effectiveness is flimsy. It could, however, serve as a nice marketing tool in a physiotherapist's office.
- **Autolytic debridement**. Here, enzymes released from injured or necrotic tissue break down the non-viable tissue, separating it from the wound bed. **It is a natural, slow process that requires moisture. But why wait if you can help the process with your scalpel?**

**So, as you can see, all the 'non-surgical' methods of debridement are either useless or just serve as an adjunct to surgical debridement.**

**I prefer to classify 'surgical debridement' into two types — 'selective' and 'non-selective'.** Others, however, describe this entity as **'sharp debridement' and divide it into two types — 'conservative' and 'surgical'** (probably because only surgeons and podiatrists are licensed to perform 'non-selective debridement'). Now, did I manage to confuse you further? But this is quite simple.

**Surgical ('sharp') debridement = removal of tissue using surgical instruments.**

- **Selective ('conservative')** = limited to removal of only non-sensate, non-viable tissue. It doesn't require anesthesia and can be performed by all wound care licensed professionals.
- **Non-selective ('surgical')** = includes debridement of the 'entire wound' including its viable sensate margins and base. It requires anesthesia. This needs the expertise of surgical professionals.

## Selective debridement

**Selective debridement is an office procedure. It is 'clean' but not sterile — there is no need for a 'sterile field'; you can use disposable, non-sterile gloves, after washing your hands, and then proceed as follows:**

- You first clean the field with your cleansing solution *d'jour*. As always, hospitals and clinics recommend using commercial wound-cleansing solutions, but saline or even boiled and cooled tap water can be just as adequate. Everyone will warn you not to use alcohol or hydrogen peroxide because of its cytotoxicity; nevertheless, being an old surgeon, I still enjoy pouring hydrogen peroxide (medical grade, 3%) on heavily infected-necrotic wounds — watching it bubble is addictive, and hemostatic...
- True, non-viable tissue is non-sensate, but the edges of the wound, and sometimes its base, are. **So, I place a generous amount of lidocaine jelly on the wound**, cover it with gauze, and wait 10-15 minutes. Commonly, some patients may still complain about pain or discomfort, but this is what it is — total anesthesia is impractical in such circumstances. Injecting local anesthesia into the inflamed tissues around the wound is more painful.
- **Next, I use a sterile blade (#10) and forceps to remove all non-viable tissue until a healthy base is exposed.** Now, when I see the base, I know how deep the wound is — is it full thickness with the subcutaneous fat exposed? Are deeper structures, such as muscle, tendon, or bone, exposed? **I pay close attention to the wound margins. It must be viable and flat to allow epidermal advancement**. I pare down any surrounding callus (a cutting disposable curette is a valuable tool), and I try to 'flatten' any *epibole* observed. **A certain amount of bleeding at the base or edges of the wound is part of the deal** — it is easily controlled by a few minutes of pressure; occasionally, a touch with a silver nitrate stick is needed — a testimony that one did a thorough job.
- **Selective debridement during follow-up encounters, once the wound appears 'cleaner' and the healing process is underway, can be much less aggressive.** Now I gently scrape the base with a blade, hoping to remove the invisible but rapidly redeveloping biofilm and produce 'bleeding micro-cuts' at the wound edge to stimulate additional inflammation.

**When is selective debridement contraindicated?**

- **There is no point in debriding wounds caused by ischemia.** In this situation, just evacuate any purulent and non-adherent necrotic matter, clean the wound, and refer/arrange for revascularization of the affected limb.

- **Dry, 'stable' eschar adherent to the wound should be left alone initially**. 'Stable' means that there are no features of infection (e.g. erythema, purulence); the eschar is not 'boggy'. Just paint the area with povidone-iodine solution to reduce the bacterial burden, then cover with a dressing. Continue monitoring the wound; once the eschar starts loosening up, you can remove it, often in stages, piecemeal. Debride immediately if infection sets in.
- **The heel fat pad is notorious for its marginal perfusion** (even if the blood supply to the foot is intact). Debridement of the stable eschar covering a heel ulcer would further expose poorly vascularized fat pad tissue, risking infection and deepening or widening of the ulcer.
- **Anticoagulation and bleeding disorders are *relative* contraindications**. However, most patients presenting to the wound care clinic are usually on some 'blood thinner'. *Cautious* selective debridement is safe with no need to discontinue any of these drugs or modify their dose. However, try not to dig too deep or wide into viable tissues unless you are confident in your hemostatic skills.
- **Do not persist with selective debridement if the wound status and patient condition warrant aggressive, non-selective surgical debridement**.

## Non-selective surgical debridement

Aggressive surgical debridement is often indicated in the following situations:

- **Infected 'deep' wounds** with surrounding cellulitis (surgeons call it a deep surgical site infection).
- Wound infection with features of **systemic sepsis**.
- **Extensive necrosis** of the wound and periwound area (■ Figure 5.2).
- Underlying **osteomyelitis** (so common in 'diabetic feet').
- Extensive **undermining** and/or **tunneling** of the wound.
- When there is a need to remove **infected hardware or mesh** from the depth of the wound.
- When the wound is '**unstageable**', meaning that you don't know how deep it is because its base is obscured by necrotic tissue.

**These procedures are performed by surgeons or podiatrists under some anesthesia, occasionally in the operating room**. The techniques used are part of basic surgical training and thus beyond the scope of this book.

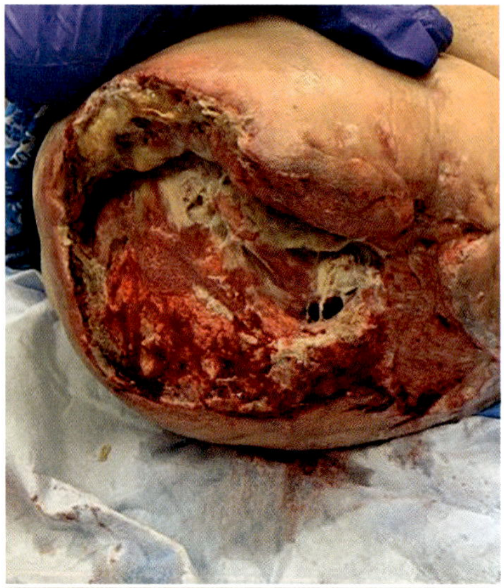

Figure 5.2. Infected, necrotic above-knee amputation stump in need of aggressive surgical debridement.

Often, I see patients with wounds 'screaming' for aggressive surgical debridement treated with yet another change of dressings or wound VAC, and yet another change of antibiotics. **So, do not procrastinate — get on board with your local surgeon, or contact the surgeon who performed the operation that resulted in the wound you are now treating**.

In the good old days, surgeons shouldered responsibility for 'their wounds' until complete healing took place. Unfortunately, these days of the prevailing 'fragmented' and allegedly 'cost-effective' care, postoperative patients are discharged as early as possible, only to present, days or even weeks later, with wound complications to their primary care provider or your wound care clinic. **Don't screw up — get the surgeon involved!**

## A few words about wound packing

**Wound packing is used to fill dead spaces in open wounds so they can heal from the base upwards, preventing premature closure of the skin and leaving non-viable or infected tissue at the base. It also provides hemostasis for freshly drained wounds**. Wound packing has already been described by the ancient Egyptians, who used lint soaked in honey for this purpose, and is practiced continuously across generations utilizing a myriad of materials.

**You can use any packing material you wish**. In the acute phase (when hemostasis is needed), I use ribbon gauze or gauze rolls (depending on the size of the wound). Subsequently, I may continue with strips cut from one of the 'modern' absorptive and/or 'medicated' materials (see ➲ Chapter 7).

**A key item: do not overpack! A common error I often observe is wounds packed too tightly — fully stuffed with packing material during subsequent changes of dressing — thus preventing filling/contraction/healing**. Yes, after initial drainage/debridement, you can pack tightly to obtain hemostasis. Still, later on, packing should be progressively 'looser' — a strip of the packing material reaching the base of the wound to serve as a wick would do the job. **Let the wound breathe and contract**.

**"If you don't produce some bleeding, you cannot claim that you did a debridement!"**

# Chapter 6

## Contamination, colonization, and infection

*An open wound is never sterile!*

In ➲ Chapter 3, I talked about the '**microbial continuum**'. You already understand that open wounds are contaminated with bacteria, but that contamination doesn't always mean infection. I also mentioned that while in theory the notion of a 'continuum' (of contamination, colonization, critical colonization, infection) appears appealing, it is less clear in practice, where 'infection' is obvious but the distinction between the first three entities is less clear, cumbersome, and often calls for an 'empirical' approach. In ➲ Chapter 4, you read about the '**assessment of infection' — the difference between 'obvious' infection and 'non-obvious infection', and about wound cultures**. Now, with all that knowledge, you are ready to read about the actual management of these entities.

### Infection

**We are now at the I of the TIME acronym (remember?)**.

**The diagnosis and treatment of infection is rather straightforward**. The local redness, swelling, tenderness, purulence, and necrosis are obvious. Surrounding cellulitis and systemic repercussions indicate that the infection is no longer 'local'. Imaging (US, CT, or MRI) could suggest involvement of deeper structures.

You manage it based on the findings: for **'local' infection**, drain, debride, culture, administer oral antibiotics, watch carefully, and re-evaluate; for 'spreading' or 'deep' infection, consider admission, i.v. antibiotics, further imaging, and call a surgeon.

**Remember**: signs of infection can be ambiguous in **immunocompromised** patients who cannot mount an inflammatory response. Also, in the **morbidly obese**, signs can be subtle or absent. A typical example is infection in **diabetic feet** — inside the swollen but otherwise harmless-looking toe, the joint and bone may be destroyed by osteomyelitis. **You must be super suspicious of these patients.**

## Contamination/colonization

I am going to repeat and re-repeat myself here and elsewhere in this book, for repetitions are crucial to 'adult learning'. **So here I go again: all open wounds harbor bacteria. If you 'poke' them with a swab and obtain a culture, it will always grow some bacteria. But most such positive cultures do not call for antibiotics; in fact, many wounds do not need to be cultured at all.**

**But this is not the prevailing practice I observe in the 'community'.** Instead, patients with non-healing wounds are started by the referring docs on oral antibiotics — "just in case" — and cultures are taken (by an inappropriate technique). Undoubtedly, in many cases, the antibiotics are unnecessary (and potentially harmful). And most cultures taken are redundant, yielding irrelevant results, which could mislead the unaware wound care practitioner into administering more unnecessary antibiotics.

Now you may say: yes, I know the wound is 'contaminated' because all open wounds are 'contaminated'. But how do I know if it isn't 'colonized' or 'critically colonized', thus potentially preventing healing?

**Let us consider, for example, a paraplegic diabetic patient with a heel ulcer you see for the first time** (■ Figure 6.1). **There are no obvious signs of infection.** You start conventional wound care, which (as discussed below) would include measures suppressing bacterial burden in the wound. In parallel, you try to control wound-related factors (e.g. local edema, repeated pressure injury) and patient-related factors (e.g. diabetes), which are likely to prevent healing. **At this time, there is no need to take cultures or consider any antimicrobial agents.**

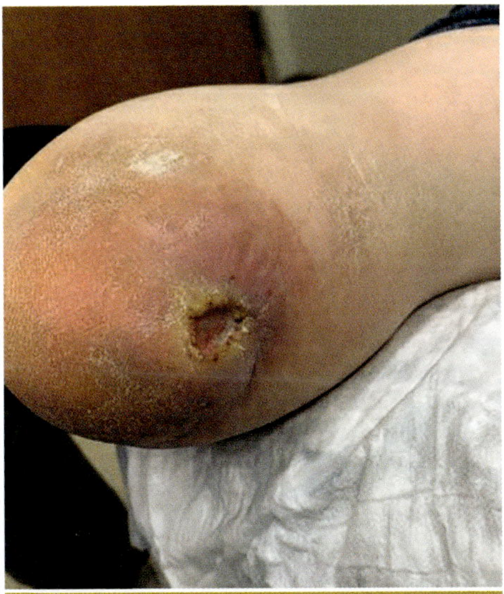

**Figure 6.1. Pressure ulcer on the heel of a paraplegic patient with an edematous foot.**

**A week later, you see the patient again**. The wound looks the same. No progress. You repeat local care, gently 'scraping' the elusive biofilm, and let occupational therapy (OT) control the leg edema better.

**A week later, the wound looks the same** — no healing activity whatsoever. The base of the wound is pale and slimy, with no granulation tissue seen. Now you should start thinking: are there too many bacteria residing in this wound, or is it colonized, stalling healing? **Now is the time to consider taking a culture.**

Preliminary results of the culture will be available within 24-48 hours. So, if you are 'worried', you could apply a local antibacterial agent empirically into the wound (e.g. mupirocin ointment 2%, which is effective against a wide range of Gram-positive bacteria). **But again: no systemic antibiotics are needed**.

## Bacteriology

■ **Table 6.1 lists the bacteria that are known to reside in chronic wounds** (fungi are rare, except in severely immunocompromised individuals, and are seldom pathogenic unless there are systemic signs).

**Table 6.1. Common wound bacteria and a common fungus.**

| | |
|---|---|
| ***Staphylococcus aureus*** | **Nearly universal presence**. Can be 'methicillin-resistant' (MRSA) |
| ***Streptococcus*** | Beta-hemolytic |
| ***Pseudomonas aeruginosa*** | Typically associated with a greenish exudate |
| ***Enterococcus*** | Mainly *E. faecalis* but other species are possible |
| ***Proteus spp.*** | |
| **Other Gram-negative bacteria** | *Klebsiella spp., Enterobacter spp., Serratia spp.* |
| **Anaerobic bacteria** | Typically, in deeper, oxygen-deprived wounds |
| ***Candida albicans*** | A fungus |

Here are a few points:

- Bacteria such as *Staphylococcus epidermidis*, *Staphylococcus aureus*, and *Streptococcus spp.* are part of **normal skin flora**. It is no wonder that they habitually contaminate open wounds.
- **In more than half of the cases, a single organism is cultured**. Multiple organisms (Gram-positive and -negative) are cultured in the rest.
- ***Staphylococcus aureus* (>90%) and *Pseudomonas aeruginosa* are the most common organisms causing infection in chronic wounds**. The latter tends to settle in the deeper part of the wound, the former more superficially — thus the sampling technique matters.
- The wound characteristics and etiology matter: 'early' superficial wounds tend to harbor staphylococci; *Pseudomonas* invades the larger, chronic wounds, whereas anaerobes tend to reside in the very deep, dark recesses — like the neglected decubitus ulcers.
- Each of these organisms can participate in forming a biofilm, arrest wound healing, enlarge it, or infect it.
- *Streptococcus* species typically spread as cellulitis. Anaerobes produce malodorous necrosis.

- **Methicillin-resistant *Staphylococcus aureus* (MRSA)**, which is endemic in some communities or acquired during previous hospitalizations, can infect chronic wounds; for example, a patient with a wound on her shin following drainage/debridement of a neglected post-traumatic hematoma. I applied mail stamp-size pieces of split-thickness skin graft on the granulating wound. It was healing rapidly until the area reddened and purulent discharge covered the wound. A culture grew MRSA. A short course of oral doxycycline and local care with mupirocin ointment cleared the wound within a few days (■ Figure 6.2).

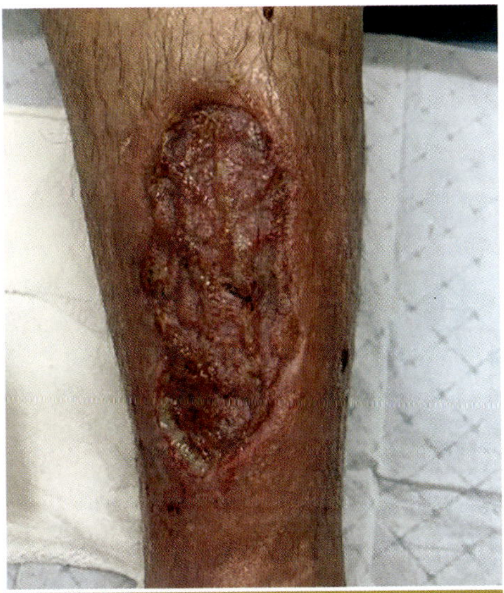

**Figure 6.2. A post-traumatic wound on the shin, covered with 'stamps' of split-thickness skin graft. The wound was infected with MRSA.**

**Now you can understand why culturing wounds plays an essential role, despite the limitations outlined above.** Because if the culture findings are clinically significant, you must know which bacteria(s) to treat and with which drugs.

**And by the way, while you can be selective in swabbing wounds which are 'not obviously infected', all 'obviously' infected wounds must be swabbed.** The most common responsible organism is indeed *S. aureus*, which is susceptible, for example, to oral doxycycline (or sulfamethoxazole-trimethoprim) or i.v. vancomycin, but what if another of the organisms mentioned above is responsible for the infection?

## Interpretation of the wound culture

How to obtain a 'reliable' wound culture was discussed in ➲ Chapter 4. As mentioned, most laboratories use semiquantitative methods, and details of reporting varies widely across the many locations where you may be practicing. **Herein I will share with you how I interpret and apply the results of *semiquantitative* wound cultures in clinical practice — emphasizing that 'nothing is written in stone', that it is not 'black and white', and that you must constantly use your judgment, correlating the lab report with the evolving clinical picture.**

**The microbiological lab submits reports in three steps:**

- Gram stain (the next morning).
- Culture results (within 48 hours).
- Antibiotic susceptibility (a day later).

### Gram stain

It reports whether any **microorganisms** are present (or absent), in what **quantity** ('rare' or 'abundant'), are they **Gram-positive** or **-negative** or both, their **morphology** (cocci or rods or both) and the presence or absence of **polymorphonuclear cells** (PMNs). All these 'items' should be considered, again, together with the clinical scenario; for example:

- **A report on 'no organisms identified' can be 'reassuring'**, whereas a 'scant' presence of bacteria hints at colonization rather than infection.
- **Gram-positive cocci in clusters** points to staphylococci, including MRSA.
- **Gram-positive cocci in pairs or chains** points to *Streptococcus* species, including *Enterococcus* species.
- **Rods** can be **Gram-negative** (e.g. *Pseudomonas*, *E. coli*, *Klebsiella pneumoniae*) or **Gram-positive** (e.g. *Corynebacterium* species, *Clostridium* species).
- The presence of **PMNs** in chronic wounds can signify a persistent inflammatory state rather than acute infection. **Their activity contributes to the 'stalled' healing by diverse mechanisms.** On the other hand, multiple PMNs and bacteria may suggest acute infection. In addition, the PMNs can be trapped in the biofilm and are thus absent in the Gram stain. Is it confusing? Yes, I know, so I pay little attention to the PMNs.

**The Gram stain is a 'preliminary step'.** It can be reassuring (e.g. no bacteria seen, a few PMNs) that there is no infection, and you can wait for the culture results; or that your empiric choice of antibiotics is correct — for example, that you have prescribed doxycycline and Gram-positive cocci in clusters are seen.

## Culture results

A few points concerning culture results:

- **It will report "no growth" or list the organism(s) cultured and its 'growth category'**. The latter will be described as "occasional growth" (+), "light growth" (++), "moderate growth" (+++) or "heavy growth" (++++).
- **The 'moderate' and 'heavy growth' indicate significant bacterial counts**, corresponding to counts greater than 100,000 per gram (>$10^5$ CFU/g) on quantitative cultures — **suggesting infection**.
- "Occasional or light growth" may represent **colonization**.
- **When over three organisms are identified, the report states: "mixed skin flora"**. In that case the lab will test for antibiotic susceptibility only on request.
- **The type of bacteria identified matters**. So, for instance, the presence of *Pseudomonas* in a chronic wound always represents some degree of infection, but *Staphylococcus epidermidis* — a common skin bacteria — is usually a 'benign colonizer'; 'usually' but not 'always' for it can take part in the formation of biofilm and in some cases be responsible for infection.
- Sometimes two or three bacteria will be reported but **only one of them is predominant and clinically significant**. Should you treat only the dominant one or all of them?

## Antibiotic susceptibility

A few points concerning antibiotic susceptibility:

- **About 3 days after the culture has been obtained, the lab reports to which antibiotics are the isolated organisms susceptible. Each drug tested is annotated with either a "S" (sensitive) or "R" (resistant).**
- **Some labs add the 'MIC dilution'** (minimum inhibitory concentration dilution) for each drug. In this test, different concentrations of the agent are placed in separate tubes to which the isolated organism is added. The tube with the lowest concentration showing no growth represents the MIC. In theory, if the organism is susceptible to a few agents, the one with the lower MIC would be the most effective.
- **Which, and how many, antibiotics are evaluated differs between locations and labs**. The lab I use reports susceptibility against 10-15

drugs. A friend from Germany showed me a copy of a report from his hospital listing 30 antibiotics. The Germans of course are known to be thorough. 😊

**Comments by labs**: some labs add comments to their reports — for example, "Mixed skin flora, suggesting contamination" or "Heavy growth of *S. aureus*, suggesting infection."

## Culture results are 'dynamic', not 'static'

So, after 3 days, you have the 'final' results of the culture. Now you must decide:

- **There is no infection or significant contamination** — continue conventional wound care?
- **Probably critical colonization** — apply an antimicrobial agent to the wound?
- **Probably infection** — administer antibiotics — orally or systemically? And which drug to use?
- **Discontinue the empiric antibiotics** started 3 days ago?
- **Change the empiric antibiotics** already started or add another agent?

Below are examples from my patients last week.

**A 91-year-old lady with a full-thickness localized burn (from a warming blanket) on the buttocks**. She declined early excision of the eschar and primary closure. I treated the wound with silver sulfadiazine cream (SSD™) awaiting spontaneous separation of the eschar. Two weeks later the eschar appeared raised and 'boggy'. I removed the eschar and cultured the murky exudate found underneath (■ Figure 6.3). **I didn't start her on antibiotics**. Here are the culture results:

- **Gram stain (same day)**: rare neutrophils, rare Gram-positive cocci in pairs, rare Gram-negative rods.
- **Growth (a day later)**: moderate *Proteus mirabilis*, light *Enterococcus faecalis*.
- **Growth and susceptibility (2 days later)**: moderate *Proteus mirabilis*, moderate *Enterococcus faecalis*, moderate *Proteus mirabilis* susceptibility — see ■ Figure 6.4.

**Only now have I started the patient on oral ampicillin, to which both bacteria were susceptible**. In the absence of clear local signs of infection, there was no need to rush and administer empiric antibiotics immediately.

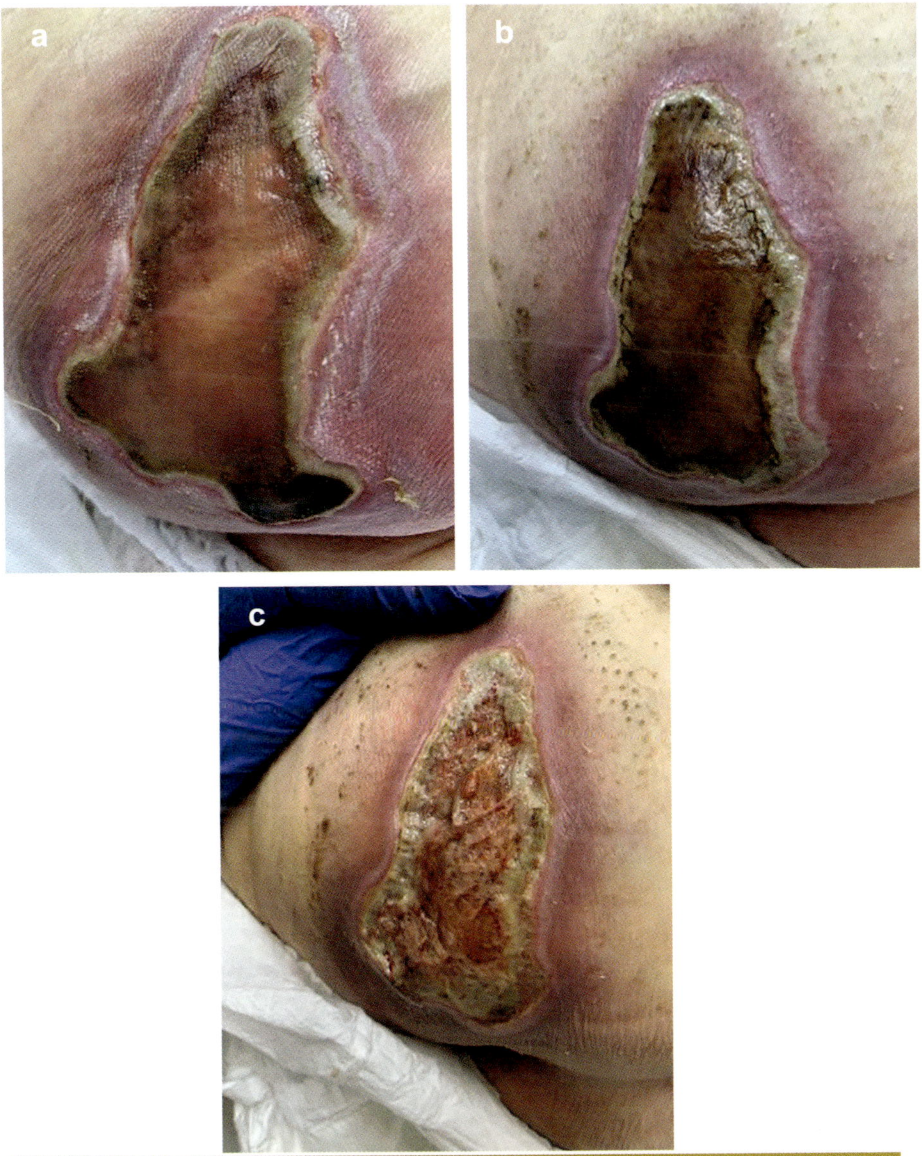


**Figure 6.3. Burn on the buttocks. a) Presentation. b) Two weeks later. c) After removal of eschar.**

Specimen Information

| | | | |
|---|---|---|---|
| Order: | Culture. Aer... | Collect Date/Time: | |
| Growth Ind: | POS | Last Update Date/Ti... | |
| Status: | Completed | Testing Site: | |
| Source: | Wound | Freetext Source: | |
| Body Site: | BUTTOCK - ... | Accession #: | |

| | Proteus mirabilis | Enterococcus faecalis |
|---|---|---|
| Drug | MIC Interp | MIC Interp |
| Ampicillin (1) | S | S |
| Cefazolin | I | |
| Cefotaxime | S | |
| Cefoxitin | S | |
| Cefpodoxime | S | |
| Ceftriaxone | S | |
| Cefuroxime/Axetil | S | |
| Ciprofloxacin | S | |
| Doxycycline | R | |
| Gentamicin | S | |
| Levofloxacin | S | |
| Penicillin | | S |
| Trimethoprim/Sulfa | S | |
| Vancomycin | | S |

**Figure 6.4. A copy of the susceptibility report on a patient's wound culture.**

**An 87-year-old man presenting with a pressure sore on his *left* heel 2 weeks after discharge from a university hospital, where he had undergone revascularization of his *right* lower extremity for critical ischemia.** (This is common in our 'modern times': each specialty focuses on the 'organ' it is managing — why check the left foot when we are treating the right lower limb? Preventive measures? Nurses are too busy with useless documentation!) Initially, I evacuated a large blister on the heel, exposing a full-thickness pressure injury (■ Figure 6.5), and started local wound care. A week later, the patient complained about increasing pain, and the entire area was very tender. I debrided it 'gently' — as mentioned above, the heel 'fat pad' is poorly vascularized and one must avoid 'aggressive debridement' — and took a swab for culture. The increasing pain and tenderness suggested infection, so I started him on 'empirical' antibiotics — doxycycline (which in our environment is highly effective against staphylococci) and applied mupirocin ointment on the wound. Here are the culture results:

- **Gram stain (same day)**: no neutrophils, no organism observed.
- **Growth (a day later)**: no growth.
- **Growth (2 and 3 days later)**: no growth.

**I did not stop the antibiotics. Yes, most likely no infection was present, but the culture results could be false-negative, and, in general, clinical findings overrule the lab results**. A week later, the pain/tenderness subsided, and the wound looked 'better'. Was it infected? Did the antibiotics help? Who knows?

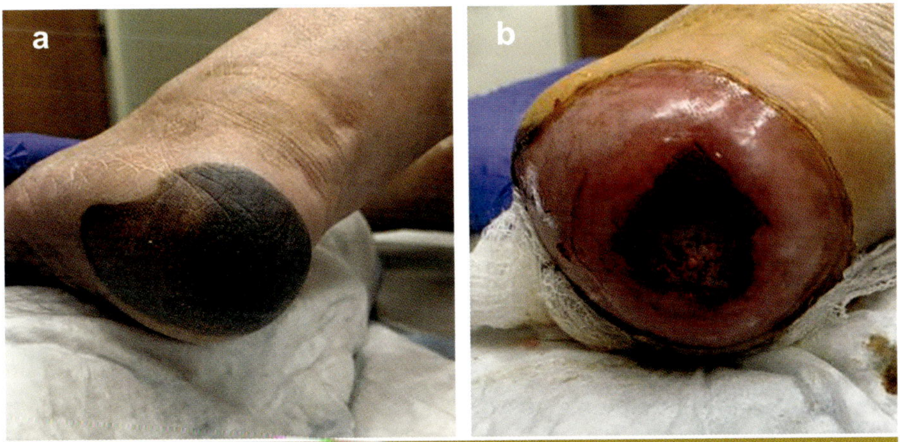


**Figure 6.5. Pressure injury to the left heel. a) On presentation. b) A week later.**

These examples show that the interpretation of wound cultures is not 'black and white'. Even for me, with many years of experience, in some instances it's more based on guesswork than on science.

**If wound care is like complex cooking, interpreting cultures is a puzzle**. Of course, you can always consult an infectious disease specialist. However, members of that specialty, in my experience, tend to overtreat…

## Anaerobic culture

What we have been talking up to now concerns 'routine' **aerobic** cultures. Cultures for **anaerobes** require different handling and are not routine, as anaerobic bacteria (which work in synergy with aerobes) tend to be found in the deeper areas of wounds and within biofilms. **Tissue biopsy or infected fluids are typically used to isolate anaerobes**.

**Suspect and look for anaerobes in the following situations**:

- Wounds resulting from gastrointestinal or gynecological operations.
- Foul-smelling discharge.
- Necrotic tissue, gangrene.
- Gas in tissues.
- Wounds associated with malignancy or other processes producing tissue destruction.
- Wounds resulting from human or other bites.

Obviously, if you seriously suspect that anaerobes have contributed to the infection of the wound, you should start treating it empirically — see the next section.

## Antibiotics

Bear with me. I will repeat some of what you read above.

**There is no doubt that, like in other fields of medicine, antibiotics are overprescribed, in an anarchic way, and administered for an excessive duration**.

> **The selection of antibiotics for proven or suspected chronic wound infection is relatively straightforward** — you should follow the **general principles** used in other fields: **know the presumptive pathogens in your environment and their susceptibility (follow local antibiograms), try to limit their use, and know when to stop them**.

The use of **topical antibiotics** applied to the wound, while attractive, is **controversial and less firmly established**. In addition, the use of **various topical non-antibiotic antimicrobial agents** (not all of them are 'classical antiseptics', but here I will discuss them under the umbrella of 'antiseptics') **continues to be practiced in chaos: each chef adding their preferred ingredients to the soup, believing it will taste better**. Here I will attempt to insert some common sense into your (and my) mind.

## Systemic antibiotics

**The 'typical' patient will arrive at your wound care clinic with some antibiotics on board, or after having finished a course (or a few courses) of this or that antimicrobial agent**. It seems that most referring docs who see an open wound, with some 'redness', feel compelled to 'do something' about it…

## Intravenous antibiotics

**We rarely use i.v. antibiotics in the ambulatory setting of the wound care clinic**. They are indicated when the infection spreads beyond the wound with features of 'sepsis' (e.g. cellulitis complicating chronic venous ulcers, deep surgical site infections, or infections associated with surgical hardware). But such patients usually need to be hospitalized, so let the hospitalists, subspecialists, and infectious disease team make the decisions. However, in some situations, patients can receive i.v. antibiotics on an ambulatory basis (e.g. a patient with an MRSA infection on his face in need of vancomycin).

## Oral antibiotics

**After reading all the above, you should have some idea of when a course of antibiotics is indicated and know the presumptive causative organisms**. Here is how I do it:

- **I usually start empirically with doxycycline**, for it covers staphylococci, including MRSA, in the vast majority of cases. And I await the culture results.
- **Based on the culture results, I may change to another drug** (e.g. to sulfamethoxazole-trimethoprim [Bactrim®]) if the MRSA cultured is susceptible to this drug but resistant to doxycycline, **or add another drug** (e.g. ampicillin) if the culture shows significant growth of *S. faecalis*. **I would ignore the culture results if the wound is improving** at early follow-up.
- ***Pseudomonas*** (a common wound pathogen) is resistant to oral antibiotics except the fluoroquinolones (ciprofloxacin, levofloxacin). It is increasingly resistant to these agents as well. **So, for 'local' infection with *Pseudomonas spp.* I prefer topical management as described in the next section**. For invasive-spreading infection, i.v. antibiotics are indicated, based on susceptibility.
- **What about anaerobes?** If I suspect infection with anaerobes (e.g. a 'smelly' deep wound), then amoxicillin/clavulanic acid (Augmentin®) is a reasonable choice; it also covers staphylococci (non-MRSA) and

some Gram-negative bacteria. Adding a classical anti-anaerobe agent such as metronidazole or clindamycin is another option.

- **Duration of administration? It depends on the type and severity of infection and the response to treatment. Typically, for a 'local' infection, I never prescribe an antibiotic for longer than a week.** Obviously, when infections are 'spreading' and/or there is a need to change drugs, longer courses may be necessary — in some cases for many weeks (e.g. osteomyelitis associated with a diabetic ulcer).

**Whatever you do, the emphasis should be on shortening the duration of the course as much as possible.** Try to reassess the situation within 72 hours, asking yourself:

- Are antibiotics truly necessary?
- Perhaps topical therapy would be sufficient?
- Should I discontinue?

**That an ER physician prescribed antibiotics for 14 days (as they commonly do) doesn't mean that the patient must complete an unnecessarily long course. Stop it!**

## Topical antibiotics

**If you can apply an antimicrobial agent directly into the wound, why not use it instead of the oral route?** And indeed, topical antibiotics immediately achieve high wound concentrations, decreasing bioburden, reducing colonization, preventing progression to infection, or treating it.

**However, compared with topical antiseptics (see below), topical antibiotics have a few disadvantages**: a significant risk of local sensitization (i.e. 'contact dermatitis') and the emergence of bacterial resistance. In addition, the spectrum of the agents used is limited (i.e. antiseptics kill *all* microorganisms, antibiotics just a few). Moreover, antiseptics are more effective at disrupting biofilms!

**Therefore, I use topical antibiotics only for short-term management (up to 2 weeks) to treat proven colonization or a local infection targeting specific bacteria. I don't use it as prophylaxis — to prevent infection.**

Here are a few pertinent points:

- **Antibiotic ointments.** Numerous agents are available, on prescription or 'over the counter'; for example, a **'triple antibiotic ointment'** (a mix of polymyxin B, bacitracin, and neomycin effective against both Gram-positive and -negative bacteria), **fucidic acid** (targeting Gram-positive organisms), **clindamycin** (anti-staphylococci and anaerobes), **gentamycin** (with its broad activity against Gram-negative bacteria as well as staphylococci), and **metronidazole**, the classic anti-anaerobe treatment. **Mupirocin** 2% is highly effective against staphylococci species (including MRSA) and *Streptococcus pyogenes*. Unfortunately, overuse has resulted in reports of increasing resistance. **Silver sulfadiazine (SSD™) cream** (the 'gold standard antimicrobial prophylaxis for burns) is active against Gram-negative and -positive bacteria, including *Pseudomonas* and staphylococci. **In my view, all the above topical agents are misused and overused chaotically. I use them sparingly.** For example, I may apply mupirocin ointment for a week or so to a 'stalled' wound that is highly colonized with staphylococci — especially MRSA. The broad-spectrum **SSD™** cream I use for early burn management and on diabetic feet. **Gentamicin ointment** I would apply on wounds heavily colonized/infected with *Pseudomonas*.

- **Antibiotic solutions**. Topical antibiotics can be diluted into solutions. **The advantage of solutions is that they can be installed in deep cavities**. I use it rarely. For example, an elderly lady, who had leukemia and was on chemotherapy, presented with a large labial abscess. I drained it and treated it with empiric antibiotics (amoxicillin-clavulanate). The large wound 'stalled' with rigid, painful margins despite repeated debridement and prolonged drainage with Penrose drains (■ Figure 6.6). Eventually, cultures grew a *Pseudomonas*. I

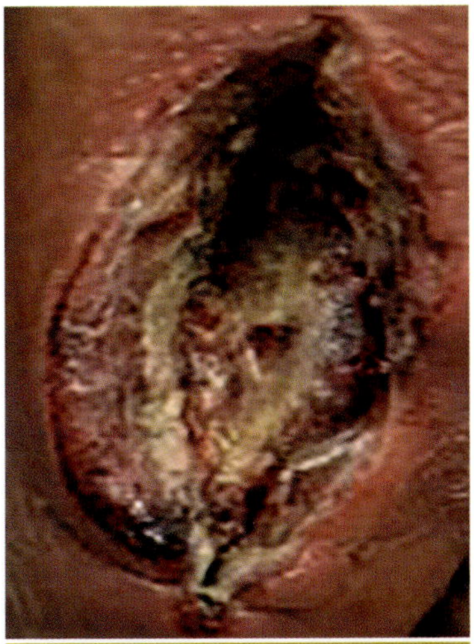

**Figure 6.6. Non-healing wound of the labia, after drainage of an abscess, in an immunocompromised patient.**

tried topical treatment with **acetic acid** (vinegar) with no success. I tried a **gentamicin** solution: gauze pads soaked in the solution were applied to the wound twice daily. Within a day, the pain subsided, and the wound began to fill in. It healed completely within 2 weeks. Ask your pharmacist how to dilute the drug for you...

## Topical 'antiseptics'

**Antiseptic agents kill not only bacteria but also other microorganisms** (e.g. fungi, yeast, and viruses). However, the aim of their use in chronic wound care is not to sterilize the wound (**remember: chronic wounds are never sterile and never can be**), but to reduce the bioburden and disrupt biofilm, thus preventing heavier colonization and infection during the prolonged phases of wound healing.

**A wide variety of antiseptic agents are used worldwide**. Even within the walls of one kitchen, each chef has his or her own favorite ingredients. In my own environment, one wound care specialist prefers silver-based products, the podiatrist likes povidone-iodine (Betadine®), whereas I love honey. In the absence of any solid evidence that one agent is 'better' than the other, it is no wonder that the chaos continues in the literature as well as in clinical practice.

There is no point discussing in detail the numerous agents available; I will mention only a few (that I use). **Whatever antiseptics you decide to use in your own setting, check whether they could be harmful to the adjacent and healing tissues in specific concentrations.**

> **The great physician William Osler (1849-1919) wrote: "Soap and water and common sense are the best disinfectants."** He may have been right: **there is nothing wrong with only soap and water. Not all wounds need elaborate wound care!**

**I use antiseptics in two main settings**:

- **The initial cleaning of a dirty/infected wound**. I prepare the area with povidone-iodine (you can dilute it if you wish), perform the debridement, and then wash the wound with **hydrogen peroxide 3%**. Some authors caution that this agent is 'highly toxic' to tissues, but, again, I like watching how the bubbles form and 'suffocate the bugs'; these bubbles help debride and clean the tissue and have a proven hemostatic effect. (**Gas emboli into the heart or brain are described as an infrequent complication of hydrogen peroxide if injected under pressure into deep cavities with the patients sitting up**.) I may repeat the 'spiel' during the subsequent encounter, if necessary.

- **'Maintenance' during wound care. Occasionally, I would use silver-impregnated products** in different commercial dressings. **Silver, a heavy metal that is an effective antiseptic, has become the most used topical antimicrobial in the USA**. The reason, no doubt, is due to the industry pressures to use expensive silver-impregnated dressings — whether indicated or not. The prolonged use of silver products can cause argyria (permanent gray discoloration of the skin), and it can delay wound healing. **Thus, I avoid using any silver-based products (including SSD™ cream) for more than 2 weeks.**
- **For 'greenish wounds' suggesting *Pseudomonas* colonization or infection, I use a 3% acetic acid solution** from our pharmacy: a gauze pad is soaked in the solution and applied daily to the wound. In a low-resource environment, this cheap and readily available antiseptic (with the addition of paraffin, it becomes an ointment) is successfully used on all sorts of wounds. For how to dilute your kitchen vinegar for such use, Google it up.

**But my favorite antiseptic agent, which I have continued using for many years, is not even a real antiseptic — it is HONEY!**

## Topical honey in wound care

**The superb wound-healing properties of honey have been appreciated for thousands of years all over the world (Egypt, India, Greece, Africa).** The ancients realized that honey never spoils — it never expires — and when placed onto dirty, stinking wounds, the smell becomes less pungent, and the wound cleans up. Of course, they did not know why — that the low moisture content of honey, its high concentration of sugar, its acidity, and production of hydrogen peroxide inhibit the growth of all microorganisms. **Later, in modern times, the antimicrobial, anti-inflammatory, and tissue-debridement effects of honey have been scientifically proven.**

**I became aware of the healing value of honey 45 years ago in South Africa** when our 'housemaid' developed an ugly-looking stasis ulcer on her leg. I debrided the ulcer, treated it with various antiseptics and lotions, and applied leg compression; it didn't heal. Then an older African lady came over from a neighboring house with some raw honey. "Try this," she said, "this is what we used in the old village." We did; the ulcer healed promptly. **Since then, I have become addicted to honey — not on my toast, but on wounds — all kinds of wounds!**

Until about 10 years ago, I used solely 'commercial' honey, bought at the local supermarket, preferring the 'creamed', thicker variety, which is easy to 'smear' into the wound and doesn't spill onto the peri-wound area. But honey is honey, and I let patients use whatever honey they can get. But one day, one of my wound-honey-treated patients was seen by a young infectious disease specialist in an 'ivory tower'. And the guy sounded an alarm: "Schein is using Walmart honey… not the medical-grade honey approved by the FDA." So, immediately, we were ordered to throw away our jars of 'commercial' honey and use the many times more expensive tubes of '**medical-grade honey**' instead.

Medical-grade honey (there are a few such products on the market) is a sterilized product made from *Leptospermum scoparium* (Manuka) honey, which is harvested only in New Zealand and Australia. **The rationale for sterilizing honey is to eliminate *Clostridium botulinum* spores that were sporadically detected in non-sterilized honey products**. However, all reported cases of botulism associated with consumption of honey occurred in infants (under the age of 12 months) after *oral* ingestion of honey, none after topical use. **There has not been a single case reported of botulism or wound infection with *C. botulinum* in adults with topical use of any honey product!** And in fact, non-medical-grade honey is widely and safely used around the world where medical-grade honey is not readily available. So, within the walls of my clinic, I use 'medical-grade honey'. **But I tell patients that at home they can use whichever honey they want — why waste so many dollars on a tiny tube of one of the 'medical-grade' products?**

**Think about it: honey is the perfect 'antiseptic' to apply to wounds**:

- It's hyperosmolar, draws fluid from the wound bed, reduces edema, and promotes autolytic debridement.
- It keeps dry wounds moist.
- It creates an acidotic environment supporting tissue repair.
- It degrades biofilm.
- It produces low-level hydrogen peroxide with its antimicrobial effect, but no cytotoxicity.
- It doesn't promote bacterial resistance.

Therefore, I use it liberally for all kinds of wounds: clean, contaminated, and infected; venous ulcers, pressure ulcers, diabetic ulcers, and so on.

**"An old mentor of mine used to say: 'You can treat the wound with anything you want — whiskey, coca cola, even urine. It doesn't matter as long as you remove all the crap from it.' It's hard to admit... but what he said makes sense."**

# Chapter 7

## Dressings

> *I describe to my students what an injured animal does: it lies under a shady bush (rest, splint) by a water source (fluids, nutrition), licks the wound frequently (debridement and moist dressing) until it is clean and healing (time and patience) — and hope it makes them think past the gorgeous dressing promoted by manufacturers' reps.*
>
> **Barry Alexander**

How true! I love this aphorism. However, when my little dachshund returns from an 'expedition' in the forest, with a deep wound on his skin, I apply creamed honey to it...

A few of my old surgical buddies laugh when I describe my wound care practice to them. To them, it all sounds nonsense. "You don't need all this BS," they say. "The main thing is debridement, then water and soap... no need for fancy dressings — just cover with some gauze. Antibiotics? Antiseptics? Wound cultures? What for? Are you crazy?"

Oh yes. Many wounds, especially the run-of-the-mill postoperative and traumatic wounds, would heal with such simple measures. **But often it's impossible to convince even experienced surgeons that chronic wounds represent a different animal altogether — how we dress them matters!**

**I admit that even for many chronic wounds, some honey and gauze will do the job — as is still practiced in less privileged environments — but in many instances, I believe, 'modern' dressings have some advantages (some true, others alleged):**

- Unlike the '4 x 4 gauze/tape methodology', the 'modern' dressings come in different sizes; some have an adhesive border sticking to the periphery of the wounds; others need a 'secondary' dressing to fix them in place — use whatever best fits the type of the wound and its location, and the condition of the surrounding skin.
- **Modern dressings facilitate 'moisture balance'**. For example, absorptive foam-based products better control exudate in productive wounds, obviating the need for frequent change of saturated dressings. At the same time, products like **hydrogels** add moisture to dry wounds.
- Some 'modern' dressings are possibly 'therapeutic' — like the **silver-impregnated** products discussed in ➲ Chapter 6, or materials coated with **collagen**.

**Are you already confused? I bet you are. For the novice entering the field of advanced wound care, the plethora of available wound care products can be confusing, overwhelming, and intimidating**. You feel like an old boy from a small town in America, familiar with two types of cheddar cheese, entering a cheese boutique in Paris with its selection of 250 cheeses.

The industry is dumping on us a vast number of products, many essentially the same, but with different names, each coming with a lengthy brochure claiming justified or unproven 'advantages' (a Google search for "wound care products" brings 343,000,000 hits). **And when you look for the 'evidence' and the 'science'**, even the self-appointed gurus in the field — those who run the various courses and certification exams and write the books — admit that the 'evidence' to support the use of product X over Y is flimsy. As I mentioned before, the numerous studies (usually funded by the 'industry') are mostly flawed. **Therefore, one should use common sense and judgment in accordance with the principles outlined above**.

**A decent wound care clinic (like mine) can function well with no more than approximately 10 types of dressings in its cupboards; 5-7 would suffice.**

## How to select the dressing for the wound

The two primary considerations are:

- How wet or dry is the wound? **Moisture balance** — see below.
- Do you want the dressings to deliver something into the wound to help it heal?

(As promised earlier, I try to avoid trade names of the products, except for a few examples. Each of you can choose from what is available in your neck of the woods.)

### Moisture balance

So now we arrive at the **M** of the **TIME acronym for wound healing — MOISTURE**.

**Hippocrates (460-377 BC)** wrote: "No wounds should be moistened with anything except wine unless the wound is in a joint. Because dryness is more nearly a condition of health, and moisture more nearly allied to disease."

**Well, I am not sure about the wine, but now we know that moist wounds heal much faster than those left dry to form a scab. In fact, a dry cell is a dead cell!** Therefore, it is tragic or comic to see referring docs still recommending to the patient "leave the wound exposed to the fresh air..."

**What are the advantages of moist wound treatment?**

- It enhances epithelial cell migration.
- It preserves growth factors and enzymes.
- It assists autolytic debridement.
- It reduces scab formation — the scab interferes with the migration of epithelial cells.
- Above all, it prevents dehydration and cell death!

**On the other hand, *excessive wetness* impedes wound healing**:

- It macerates the skin around the wound (periwound), breaking it down, increasing its size.
- It provides an ideal environment for microorganisms.
- It slows cell migration.
- It prolongs the inflammatory phase, preventing the proliferative phase from taking over (remember ➲ Chapter 3?).

- It saturates the dressings, lifting them from the wound, flooding the periwound areas, soiling garments, causing the patients distress, and requiring frequent changes of dressing.

**Clearly, a BALANCE is needed: the wound should not be dry or wet — it must be MOIST. And this is the key to selecting dressings.**

## Wet wounds

**Excessively wet-productive wounds are common.** Think about a deep, neglected sacral bedsore, or the stasis ulcer in a swollen leg, constantly dripping tissue fluid. **Such wounds need an absorbent dressing.** There are three options that I use:

- **Alginate dressings.** These are made from pressed seaweed fibers and are highly absorbent. They retain shape and strength under high exudate levels. **The alginate product I use is Silvercel®. The sheet should extend beyond the wound margins to keep the periwound dry.** (For the choice of secondary dressings see below.) **Occasionally, I cut it into strips and insert it into deep or tunneling wounds to serve as absorbing wicks.**
- **Hydrofiber dressings.** These come 'plain' (**Aquacel®**), or — if you want to add an 'antimicrobial effect' — you can get them combined with silver (**Aquacel® Ag+**), or honey (**Aquacel® medihoney**), or even silver and calcium (it is claimed that the addition of calcium has a hemostatic effect). They form a soft gel that conforms to the wound bed. They come without sticky borders, so they need a secondary dressing to keep them in place.
- **Foam-based dressings.** These contain highly absorbent foam made from a foamed polymer, such as polyurethane, and provides cushioning as well. I use **Mepilex®**. This is a 'bordered' foam with a silicone border that gently adheres to the wound periphery. It comes in all sizes and can be used as a primary dressing (excellent for bedsores) or as a secondary dressing. A version containing silver (Ag) is available.

## Moist wounds

**When the wound is 'moist', all you need to do is prevent it from drying out.** Most wounds will reach the 'moist' state at some stage. Here, **occlusive dressings** avoid moisture loss and facilitate autolytic debridement. There are many options to choose from, tailored to the wound's characteristics. For example:

- A **hydrocolloid (e.g. DuoDERM®)**: this is a self-adhesive patch which adheres to the periwound but not to the wound's surface; it absorbs exudate from the wound, forming a soft gel which maintains moisture. I find it useful on some pressure wounds, where it protects the adjacent skin.
- **Transparent adhesive dressings (e.g. Tegaderm™ and Opsite®)** are semi-occlusive — maintaining moisture by trapping exudate while allowing air and moisture exchange. They are suitable for minor shallow wounds, and I don't remember ever using them in the wound care clinic.
- As discussed above, honey attracts and retains moisture in the wound. And honey is my preference: **a healthy dose of honey, covered with whatever you wish (even gauze) will keep the wound moist and happy**.

## Dry wounds

It is relatively rare for patients to present to the wound care clinic with a dry wound, except when the wound is covered with a dry scab. How can we add moisture to the wound?

- **Hydrogel dressings** are composed of 90% water suspended in a gel. They are advocated as 'donors' of water to dry and necrotic wounds. I am not offering an example of a product because I have never used one.
- **Xeroform™** — a gauze dressing impregnated with petrolatum and bismuth tribromophenate (preventing bacterial growth). It adds moisture to the wound, is non-adherent, and requires a secondary dressing. I like using it on healing burn sites.
- **Honey!** See ➲ Chapter 6…

## Do you want the dressings to deliver something into the wound to help it heal?

We already mentioned in ➲ Chapter 6 the various compounds included in the dressings (e.g. silver) or that can be added to it (e.g. SSD™ cream). The primary function of these compounds is to reduce the bacterial burden in heavily contaminated wounds and should not be used indiscriminately.

Prolonged use of silver dressings can lead to bacterial resistance, skin discoloration, and, rarely, toxicity. **Thus, I use it for a short term only: a week or two, and stop when the wound is clearing up.** Be particular about what you put on the wound: use the 'basic' Aquacel® rather than the more expensive Aquacel® Ag+, if there is no need for the silver.

## Do you want to use gimmicks?

As the industry continues to come forward with a steady stream of alleged magic bullets for wound care, you will be pestered by reps trying to sell you one or more of these super-expensive items. They hand out glossy brochures, describing the advantages of their product. Some of your friends may try a particular product and tell you how "wonderful it is".

**Let's take a look, for instance, at one popular item — the collagen dressing products.** They come in various formats, including sheets, powders, particles, gels, sponges, films, and pastes; some are impregnated with silver. The rationale for their use is that collagen is integral to healing by providing a scaffold for cell migration, supporting new tissue growth, and promoting epithelization. AI machines (e.g. Perplexity or Copilot) tell us that "collagen products demonstrate moderate evidence of effectiveness… improving healing rate", citing a single meta-analysis (published in some obscure journal from China) of 11 studies, from 8 countries, each including, on average, about 60 cases. **However, the same AI machines admit that "many trials are funded by collagen product companies or involve researchers with industry ties…" and criticize the "unclear randomization methods, small sample size and selective outcome reporting."**

There is a multitude of additional 'biological dressings' floating around. For example, products derived from amniotic membrane, stem cell dressings, growth factor-enriched dressings, and others. All such products boast effectiveness in healing chronic wounds based on some 'meta-analysis'. I don't have any personal experience with any of it, and frankly, I am skeptical.

**What I am trying to tell you is this: don't be a sucker. Don't start using any of the 'fancy/novel' products before looking at the evidence — not the 'evidence' presented to you by the industry, but the real one, which usually does not exist. When I watch someone shoving a piece of one of those products (XXX $ per day) into an 'unhealable' wound, I roll my eyes…**

More on wound care gimmicks in ➲ Chapter 12.

## Periwound and secondary dressings

**The management of the periwound** (the skin surrounding the wound) and the use of **secondary dressings** require a synergistic approach, and thus I will discuss them under one heading.

**The integrity of the periwound is essential for wound healing**, providing the right environment for epithelial migration and wound contraction. **However, the periwound is prone to damage from multiple factors**: maceration from wound exudate, sweat, or fistula output; tape used to secure dressings; excessively tight compression; improper placement of negative pressure wound therapy (NPWT); contact dermatitis from various topical agents, etc.

**Secondary dressings serve several functions**: they secure the primary dressing in place (e.g. when the primary dressing is not self-adhesive); they help manage moisture by catching excess secretions; and they cushion the wound against external trauma and pressure.

**How to maintain a healthy periwound?**

- For dry skin, apply a moisturizing cream.
- Avoid excessive moisture by using proper absorbent dressings and changing them as often as necessary. **The absorptive dressing should extend well beyond the wound's margins.**
- Many options are available to prevent periwound maceration. I like zinc-based ointments (like zinc oxide used for baby rash).
- For contact dermatitis, apply a steroid ointment.
- When using NPWT, I like to protect the wound edges with strips cut from a sheet of Stomahesive® (the material used to fix bags over stomas) or with Stomahesive® paste.

**Choice of secondary dressing:**

- **Use only if needed**. Many of the 'modern' primary dressings have adhesive borders (e.g. Mepilex®) or are self-adherent (e.g. DuoDERM®).
- **Location of the wound matters**. So, self-adherent foam dressings would be perfect for a pressure wound on the buttocks, but not for a wound on the heel. A gauze wrap is an excellent solution for the heel, the elbow, other mobile areas, or when you don't want to use adhesive tape directly on the skin.
- Some people's skin do not tolerate 'regular' tapes. Here we use one of the silicone-based tapes, which is kinder on the skin.

- **A compression dressing** (e.g. Unna boot) often serves as a secondary dressing.
- **When the leg wound is extremely wet/leaking**, I 'sandwich' a large absorbent pad (e.g. 'ABD' pad) between the primary and secondary dressings.

## How frequently should dressings be changed?

**The 'correct' answer would be, as *frequently* as needed, or as *infrequently* as possible to avoid disturbing the healing process. But essentially, it depends on the wound and the dressings used**:

- **'Dirty' wounds** in need of repeated debridement require frequent dressing changes.
- **Dressing 'wear time'** depends on the quantity of wound exudate they must absorb. In this respect, 'modern', absorbent dressing material (e.g. foams) has a clear advantage over the outmoded gauze/tape type of dressings.
- **The interval between dressing changes usually becomes longer as wound healing progresses**. Once you do not need to repeatedly debride, once the wound becomes less productive (look at the dressings when you remove them!), there is no need to continue disturbing it. **Let it granulate! Don't traumatize the migrating epidermal cells**. Thus, I am repeatedly surprised by patients discharged from some hospitals with instructions to change the dressing twice a day.
- **In my practice: the average frequency of dressing change is every other day. In some cases, when no one is at home to change the dressings, I bring them back to the clinic every 3 days. When compression dressings are used (e.g. an Unna boot), I may leave the primary dressing in place for 5-7 days — or even longer**.

## Additional things to consider

- **Wound bed preparation**: before changing any dressing, the wound should be cleansed appropriately and, if necessary, debrided — remember the biofilm! In the clinic, we use a commercial wound cleanser, but at home, there is nothing wrong with rinsing the wound with running tap water.
- **Always look at the edges of the wound**: it must be healthy and flat to allow epithelial advancement (**represented by the 'E' in the TIME**

**acronym of wound management**). If not, you have to apply your blade…

- **Patient comfort**: it is crucial to minimize pain during dressing changes. Moist dressings peel off easily, but **if the dressing has dried up (due to inadequate moisture balance), you should wet it thoroughly before removal. A healthy soak with saline or peroxide helps**.

**"Whatever you do, reassess frequently. If the wound is not improving within 1-2 weeks, then you must ask yourself why, and change course. Rotating the available options may be advantageous. Be creative rather than dogmatic."**

# Chapter 8

## Compression

*Swollen edematous tissues do not heal!*

Hitherto, we have covered the four elements of the TIME acronym of wound management (**T**issue, **I**nfection, **M**oisture, **E**pithelial advancement). **Unfortunately, the TIME acronym lacks a 'C' — for compression**; **for compression is essential in the management of most wounds affecting the lower extremities, where, I believe, it is almost as important as debridement and dressings**. I am repeatedly astounded how often this crucial step is neglected not only by patients — understandably, as explained below — but also by their doctors. For example, I see patients who have undergone a coronary artery bypass graft (CABG), being sent home with dehisced/necrotic wounds on their grossly edematous legs, without any compression.

**That compression, combating venous hypertension, is the key to the healing of venous/stasis ulcers, has been known for hundreds of years. But compression is also crucial in the management of *all* types of lower extremity wounds. Remember — swollen cells, edematous tissues, do not heal! And tissue swelling commonly accompanies leg wounds and wounds of all sorts: postoperative wounds, post-traumatic wounds, and particularly the 'stasis' wounds in the morbidly obese. Compression is almost always indicated!**

## Physiology of compression

Compression reduces edema by displacing the tissue fluid back into the central circulation. **The pressure applied must be graduated — higher distally and lower proximally** — to facilitate blood and lymph flow back into the heart. The effects are:

- **Reduction in venous hypertension** — counteracting the cause of the venous/stasis ulcer.
- **Control of edema** — diminishing fluid leakage from wounds.
- **Improved microcirculation** — increasing oxygen delivery to the wound.
- **Alleviating pain and discomfort**.

The compression pressure is measured in mmHg. The specific indication for compression and the patient's tolerance to it determine the pressure applied. **But in practice, the pressure exerted is empirical**.

## Spectrum and compliance

**Like with dressings, the choice of compression systems is immense**. Just go to Google and enter "compression garments for legs", and you will get almost 3 million results. The industry offers an astounding variety of choices: one-layer, multi-layer, generating a spectrum of pressures; different materials and lengths — short, long, rigid, soft, sleeves, wraps, self-adhesive, Velcro, pneumatic, with a zipper, all colors. It is not only confusing to the patient but also to the novice providing wound care. **But let us try to follow the KISS principle (keep it simple stupid)**...

**Many patients hate their compression garments**; thus, compliance with them is generally poor and decreases over time — you will see patients with beautifully healed venous ulcers return with a recurrent ulcer after they stop using compression. **There are a few reasons for poor compliance**:

- **Application difficulty**: many patients (the old, debilitated, obese) find the garments hard or impossible to put on.
- **Discomfort**: pain, itching, sweating, under the garments.
- **Skin problems**: skin irritation and pressure sores can make wearing the garments unbearable.
- **Aesthetics and lifestyle**: this applies mainly to younger patients with active lifestyles.

- **Cost**: the cost of the garments varies widely, and so does the reimbursement by various insurance companies. Who wants to spend 50 bucks on a new pair of compression stockings when a pack of cigarettes costs 10 bucks and a new iPhone a thousand?

When selecting the appropriate compression method for each patient, we must keep these factors in mind; for example, the optimal compression pressure for patients with chronic venous stasis is 30-40mmHg. But as most patients are unable to apply and tolerate such tight garments, I compromise with a lower pressure of compression, following the dictum: **any compression is better than no compression**.

## Types of compression

There are several types of compression garments, bandages, socks, stockings, or systems — the nomenclature reflects the chaos. **Herein, I will focus on the types of compression used during the 'acute phase' of wound healing. 'Maintenance compression' to prevent recurrence, after the wound is healed, will be mentioned at the end**.

### Compression to achieve wound healing

**Essentially, there are two types: 'short stretch' and 'long stretch'. I find these terms odd and prefer to call them what they really are: 'non-elastic' and 'elastic' — as outlined below**:

- **Non-elastic compression**: provides a constant, fixed compression. **Pressures are low when the patient is resting, but when the patient walks, and his muscles contract against the fixed 'envelope', the pressures increase significantly**. Naturally, pressures are lower in the morning after a night's rest but rise gradually during the day as the legs swell against the resistance. **This type of compression is ideal for ambulatory patients**.
- **Elastic compression**: stretches during walking, providing more or less constant pressure that can feel tight during the day. **This type of compression is usually preferable in sedentary patients**.
- **Combined non-elastic and elastic compression**: some 'multi-layer' systems combine both elements. **They are proven to be more effective than single-layer compression in reducing swelling and improving healing rates, and are more absorptive and thus my first choice** (as described below).

## Contraindications to compression

Before we discuss specific compression systems, let's mention when compression should be avoided or used with caution. There are a few situations:

- **Peripheral arterial disease. Of course, you don't want to compress an ischemic leg, further reducing arterial blood flow.** As mentioned in ➲ Chapter 4 and further detailed in ➲ Chapter 15, you must ensure that the leg and foot are well perfused before compressing them. **When foot pulses are not palpable, obtain ABI measurements. When the ABI is >0.8, you can compress. When the ABI is between 0.5 and 0.8, compress 'lightly' (I use a tubular knitted sleeve such as Tubigrip®). When the ABI is <0.5 — no compression!** (Get a CT angiogram and consult a vascular surgeon.)
- **Acute infection. Infections should be eradicated or controlled before proceeding with applying compression systems.** Drain and debride the infected wound, provide antibiotics, dress appropriately, and elevate the limb. For cellulitis, administer antibiotics and elevate the limb. In both situations, a 'light' temporary compression can be applied and reapplied between daily inspections of the extremity (e.g. Tubigrip®). **After a few days, when you decide there is no need to inspect the wound and the cellulitis is regressing, you can apply your compression system of choice.**
- **Decompensated heart failure.** Surely, you don't want to push fluid from the legs into the systemic circulation, further overloading a failing heart. **Start with minimal compression. Talk to the patient's cardiologist.**

## Compression systems I use in the wound clinic

Some of the patients already arrive with a compression garment (often in their pockets and not on their aching legs) — either old, stretched-out, and soiled 'graduated' stockings or some kind of wraps. I tell them to put it away; "let us first heal your leg and then we will fit you with adequate compression for long-term use at home."

**In the acute stage, I prefer to use the more effective multi-layer systems.** Quite a few such systems are available, but to simplify purchasing, and considering the restricted storage space, I use the following options consistently:

- **Profore®**. This is a four-layer, **elastic long-stretch system (thus suitable for sedentary patients)** that provides ~40mmHg at the ankle and ~17mmHg at the knee. The first layer is soft, absorbent cast padding, the second is a light support bandage, the third is a light compression bandage, the fourth is a flexible, self-adherent bandage (like Coban™). **I apply it over the 'primary' dressing, which covers the wound/ulcer. For the very 'wet' wounds, I 'sandwich' one or two 'ABD pads' in between the layers. It is perfect for those hugely swollen, constantly weeping wounds associated with venous stasis.** After a few days of compression, the happy patient returns with a dry, half the original circumference, leg. **I let the patient wear the system for up to 7 days, depending on the need to re-evaluate the underlying wound, the amount of exudate, and the patient's tolerance to the fairly 'tight' compression.** And indeed, some patients complain about excessive tightness and need the system taken down and reapplied in a 'less tight' fashion. After a week or two, when edema and weeping have greatly improved (with the help of diuretics), I switch to a more 'tolerable' compression option.
- **Unna boot. This is a 'non-elastic' (rigid) system better suited to ambulatory patients.** The so-called 'boot' was described by the German dermatologist Paul Gerson Unna (1850-1929) more than 100 years ago. **The 'basic' version consists of a long wrap of cotton gauze, impregnated with zinc oxide paste, mixed with other 'soothing' agents, such as glycerin or calamine.** When applied wet, from the toes to the below-knee level, and allowed to dry, it stiffens (within a few hours) along the contour of the leg, forming a semi-rigid, firm but flexible, cast (i.e. 'non-elastic/short stretch') which provides intermittent compression when the muscles are active. Zinc oxide offers anti-inflammatory and skin-protective properties; compression helps venous return and reduces swelling; together, they maintain a moist environment, promoting healing. **These days, the 'basic' single-layer 'boot' is supplemented with additional layers, including an 'elastic long stretch' bandage offering additional compression, available in commercial ready-to-use kits.** The kit I use consists of three layers: a zinc oxide gauze roll, an absorbent cast padding, and an elastic (Coban™-like) bandage (■ Figure 8.1). **That the Unna boot has been used for so many years shows how effective it is in numerous situations (venous ulcers, stasis dermatitis with cellulitis, any wounds associated with severe limb swelling), and thus it is my favorite compression method in the**

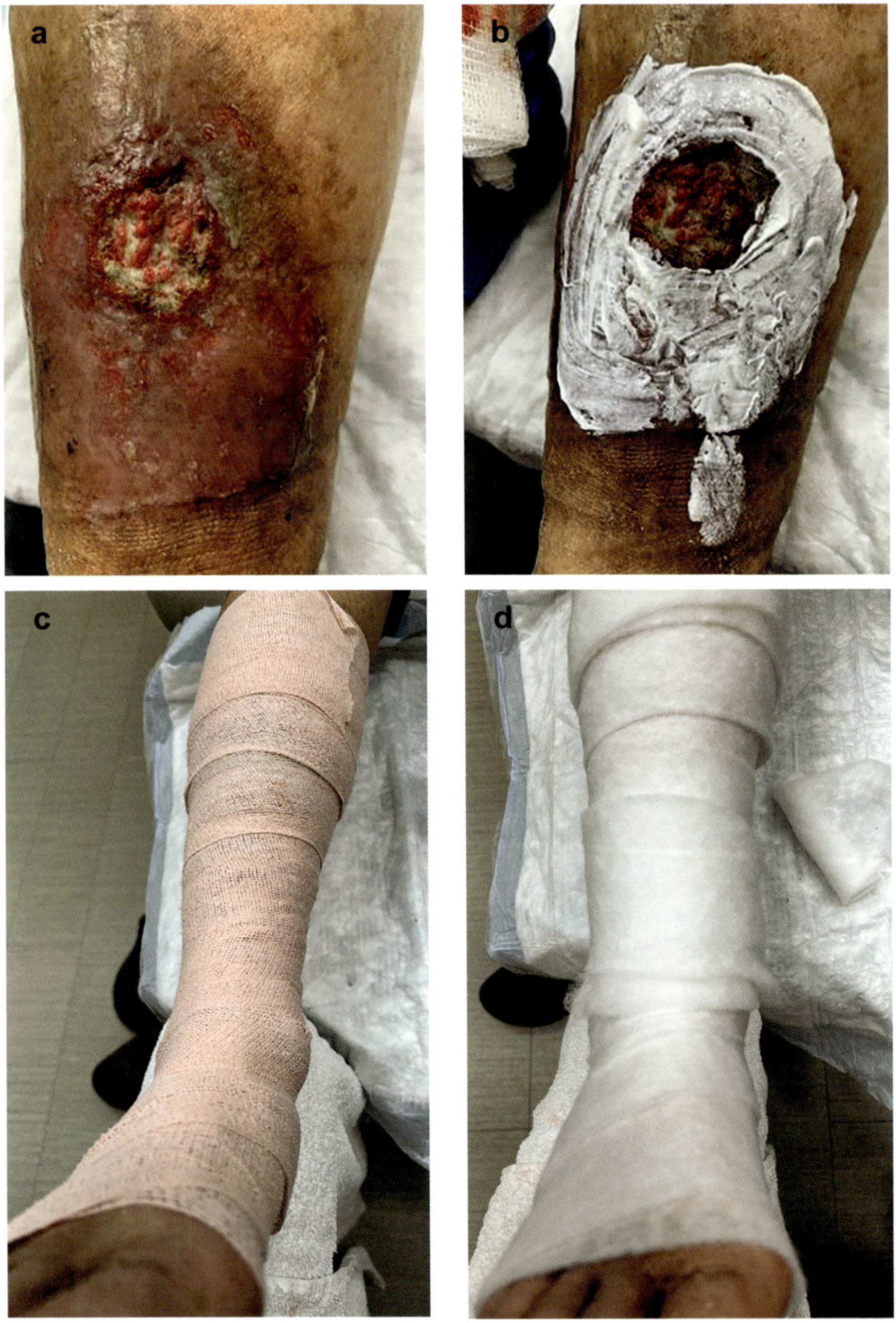


*Continued overleaf*

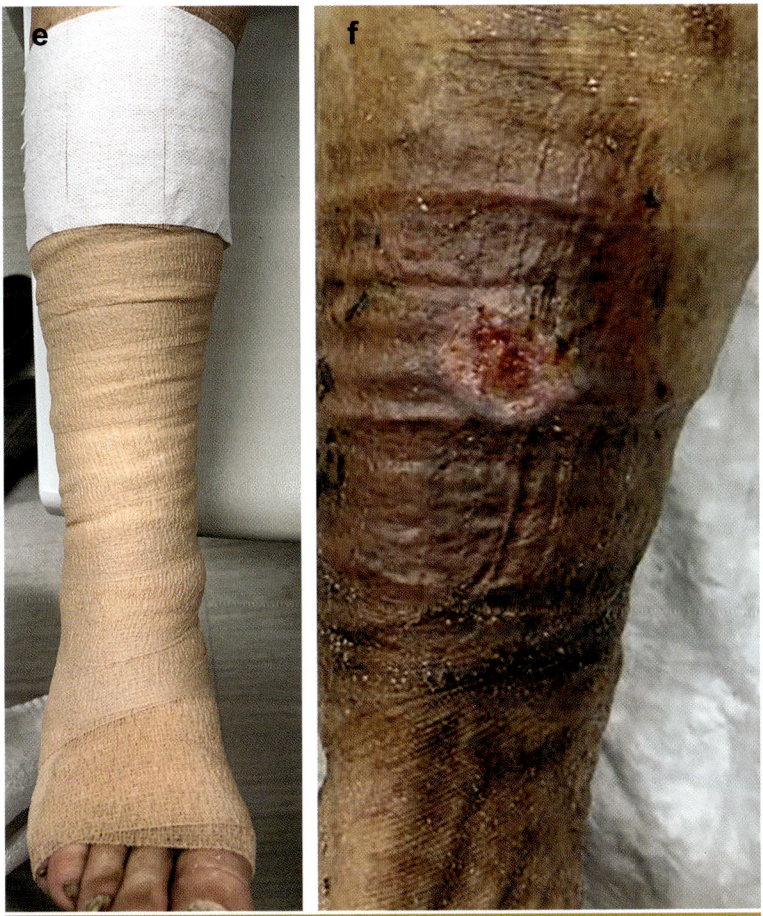


**Figure 8.1. A three-layered Unna boot used for a venous stasis ulcer. a) Venous stasis ulcer at presentation. b) Zinc paste applied on the macerated periwound. c) Zinc oxide gauze roll. d) Cast padding. e) Elastic bandage. f) The ulcer after 4 weeks of wearing the Unna boot.**

**'acute and subacute settings'**. It is cheap, easily applied, and well tolerated. **I use it predominantly in ambulant patients, but the elastic component makes it effective also in sedentary ones**.

- **Setopress®**. Unlike the Unna boot or Profore®, which are left *in situ* for up to a week (occasionally longer), and require a trip to the clinic, **this 'elastic long stretch' compression bandage is easily removed and reapplied frequently, even by the patient's family at home**. It has a printed visual guide: color rectangles that become squares when the correct extension is used. Stretching the brown rectangles to squares provides 40mmHg at the ankle; when the

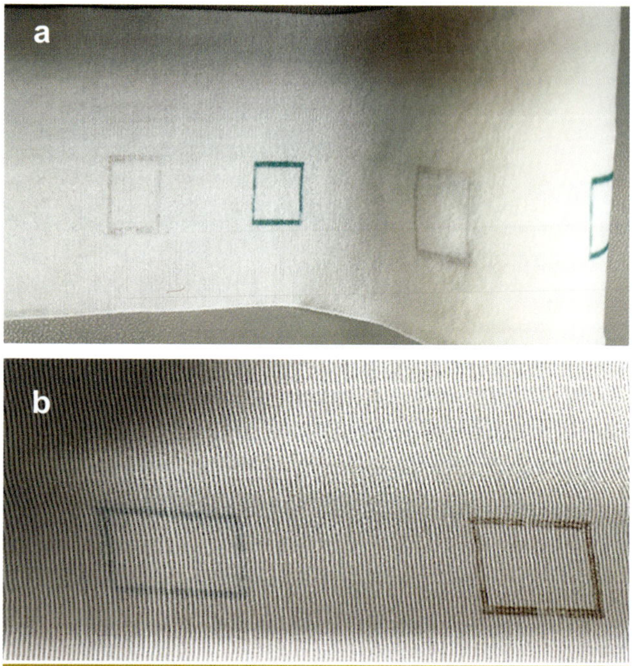


**Figure 8.2. Setopress®: note the color rectangles turning squares to indicate the desired compression pressure.**

green rectangles are stretched to squares, the pressure at the ankle is 30mmHg (■ Figure 8.2). **However, this bandage is not self-adherent and needs to be taped down at its proximal, below-knee end; hence, it tends to slip down. So, we came up with a solution**: a double length of Tubigrip® is measured and applied up to the below-knew level (the distal half-length hanging down the foot); the Setopress® is then applied over the Tubigrip®, and finally, the lower, redundant half of the sleeve is folded over the Setopress® from the toes and secured at the below-knee level.

- **Tubigrip®. This is not a multi-layer system, but it is easy to apply, versatile, washable, and cheap** (a roll of 10 meters for around 30 bucks). It is made from cotton with elastic threads. It can be cut to length and applied in a single layer or folded back into two layers. It comes in various sizes — I use the smallest, which fits comfortably. The amount of compression provided depends on the sleeve size and is around 10mmHg for a single layer and up to 30mmHg for a double layer. **It is a rare patient with a lower extremity wound who leaves my clinic without at least a Tubigrip® on their leg**. Even patients with a low ABI (but no critical limb ischemia requiring revascularization) will tolerate a single-layer large-size Tubigrip®. **As I said, some compression is better than none!**

## Compression: a few practical points

Applying any of the above compression methods may seem like a 'piece of cake', but please do not delegate it to undertrained or unsupervised individuals. **A faulty application causes harm rather than benefit.** In fact, I enjoy doing it myself. You can too!

**So, here are a few practical points**:

- Be sure that the infection is controlled, and the wound is well debrided.
- Decide which primary dressing should be applied to the wound. Again, moisture control under the compression is crucial to avoid skin maceration.
- Make sure the leg is clean and dry. Apply a moisturizing cream to dry skin. A thin layer of topical steroids will prevent itching.
- Apply with the leg elevated, the foot flexed at 90°.
- Wrap the layers of the system spirally from the toes to below the knee.
- I use a 50% overlap for each layer applied, including the first (zinc oxide) layer of the Unna boot.
- Avoid wrinkles by smoothing out each layer to ensure even tension to avoid injury to the underlying skin. This is particularly crucial when applying Unna boots.
- Provide adequate padding over bony prominences (e.g. the malleoli) to prevent pressure injury.
- Ensure that the top of the wrap is well secured to prevent slippage and a localized tourniquet effect.
- Let the patient stand up and walk (if he can) and tell you if it's not too tight.
- Instruct the patient to elevate their legs at home when the compression feels too tight; this is likely to happen at the end of the day.
- Tell them to report back immediately if the toes become painful, numb, or blue.
- What about showers? I advise wrapping the leg with a large plastic garbage bag.
- **How long can you leave the compression system in place?** If there is no need to expose the wound, you can keep it as long as it lasts. The Profore® tends to loosen and slip down after 5-7 days, but a well-

applied Unna boot can last 'forever'. I remove and reapply it every 7-10 days. I have a few non-compliant patients who keep the boot on for up to a month… with no problems!

## Maintenance compression

**Now that the wound has healed, it's your responsibility to ensure patients continue to wear compression to prevent recurrence**. And most of these patients do need 'maintenance compression': those with venous ulcers, the morbidly obese with chronic stasis dermatitis, the diabetic feet with swollen legs, etc. **Remember: swelling of the legs and feet can lead to skin breakdown. It should be prevented.**

Telling the patient, "Go back to your old compression stockings" or "go buy a new pair" is doomed to failure. **You must help the patient select the compression system that is best suited to them**; for example, graduated compression stockings, providing 30-40mmHg, are classically recommended for patients with various stasis ulcers. But most patients find it challenging to put on such 'tight' stockings. **In that case, you should help them find an alternative, as a wide range is available. For example**:

- **Ready-to-wear prefabricated socks** or sleeves of all sizes (and colors), providing a range of compression pressures.
- **Traditional graduated stockings with a zipper** for easy donning.
- **Adjustable Velcro compression wraps**, easily wrapped over the extremity, adjusting the tightness as the circumference changes. **(Note: Velcro compression garments are marketed separately for the legs and feet. Applying the leg part alone can produce severe swelling of the feet. Ensure that the patient gets and wears both parts!)**
- **Pneumatic compression machines ('lymphedema pumps')**, applied once or twice a day, can be valuable in refractory cases.

**Find out what is available in your neighborhood's shops. Some medical equipment companies provide custom-fit stockings or wraps. Search online — a wide range of attractive options is available.**

**Whatever product you choose, it must compress from the toes to the knee level. I see patients with fancy wraps applied to the leg only, with their feet ballooning out.**

**During one of the follow-up encounters, when the wound appears to be on the mend, you should consult the patient about which**

**'maintenance' compression option from the list above to get, and which size.** To estimate the correct size, you measure the circumference of the narrowest point at the ankle, the widest part of the calf, and the distance from the base of the foot (the floor) to the bend behind the knee. Then consult the sizing chart that comes with the specific product, which is always available online. Measurements should preferably be obtained during the morning hours, when leg swelling is minimal.

> **"Before discharging the patient with the healed wound from follow-up, let them bring along the new compression garment. Make sure that they (or their partner) can apply it easily and correctly. Emphasize that compression should be worn during all active hours of the day (removed at night), that the legs should be elevated when resting, and that following your advice is the absolute key to preventing recurrence!"**

# Chapter 9

## Negative pressure wound therapy (NPWT) or VAC (vacuum-assisted closure)

*Clean it, suck on it, seal it — to heal it.*

**Negative pressure wound therapy (NPWT) or vacuum-assisted closure (VAC) has revolutionized the management of 'complex' wounds. The emphasis here is on 'complex' wounds — the majority of the wounds you will have to deal with do not need to be treated with any VAC device!**

In simple terms, a 'wound VAC' is a device that helps the wound heal by applying negative pressure, namely suction. The concept is not entirely new — it has been known for a thousand years that evacuating pus and other secretions from the depth of the wound accelerates healing. It is why animals lick their wounds, and why we surgeons insert drains in wounds and/or pack them with gauze. But the use of suction or 'negative pressure' for this purpose is relatively new. The literature suggests that the concept was invented in Argentina in the early 1990s. However, the first published report of the use of suction to treat open (abdominal) wounds was by my colleagues and myself in 1986 (Schein *et al*, *British Journal of Surgery*, 1986; 73: 369-70).

As always, the medical industry rapidly jumped on the bandwagon, producing lucrative VAC devices and pushing and expanding its use across a wide variety of wound-related situations.

### How NPWT works

**The commercial wound VAC systems are typically applied in layers:**

1. A porous sponge is inserted into/onto the wound.

2. A transparent, adhesive, airtight barrier is applied over the sponge and the periwound skin.
3. An adhesive pad attached to suction tubing is placed over a hole made in the adhesive barrier.
4. The suction tube is connected to a portable vacuum pump, which generates a negative pressure of 125mmHg. The pump includes a disposable canister that collects the exudate sucked out of the wound.

**NPWT offers a few benefits**:

- It reduces swelling and inflammation by removing excess fluids from the wounds.
- It maintains moisture and protects the wound from contamination.
- It increases blood flow to the wound, thus promoting granulation and healing.
- It pulls the wound edges together, reducing its size.
- It requires a less frequent change of dressings, which is less painful and more convenient for the patient.

## Who are the candidates for a wound VAC?

**There is no doubt that NPWT, when indicated and used properly, can dramatically accelerate wound healing**. In fact, it can heal wounds that previously would have needed prolonged manipulations and multiple interventions. Nevertheless, this fantastic innovation is not required for the majority of cases you treat in your wound care clinic. **So, what are the real indications for its use?**

- **Deep, productive cavities** that would take ages to close spontaneously. The emphasis is on *deep* and *productive*! For example: the horrendous pressure sore on the buttocks; the dehisced, deeply gaping, abdominal wound in the obese patient; the large cavity with undermined skin edges resulting from drainage of a post-traumatic hematoma; the dehisced wound following spine surgery (■ Figure 9.1).
- **A dehisced, ugly, productive amputation stump**.
- **A productive deep sinus**. Here, the VAC can avoid the need for exploration/excision of the sinus.
- **A wound cavity with significant undermining of the skin edges**; the VAC obviates the need for excising additional skin and thus enlarging the wound.
- **A 'tunneling' wound**; the VAC avoids the need to unroof the tunnel to achieve healing.

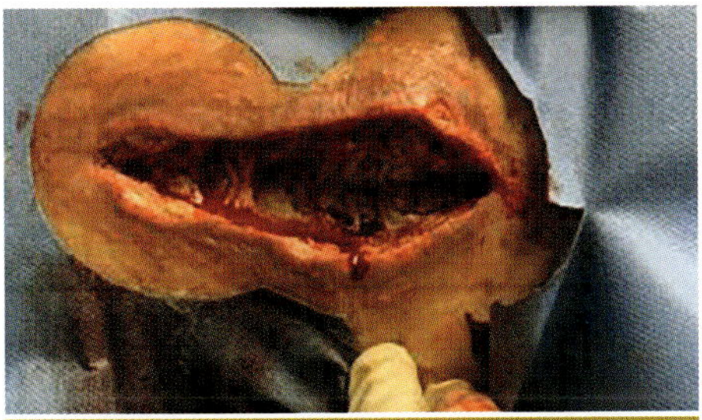

Figure 9.1. Dehisced wound on the back after spinal surgery to be managed with NPWT.

**Now you should understand which wounds *do not* need NPWT**. And, of course, the prophylactic use of VAC systems on 'fresh', primarily closed surgical wounds, which is advocated by the 'industry', is no more than an unproven gimmick!

## Contraindications to the use of NPWT

**You must avoid using the VAC system under the following situations**:

- **Infection of the wound**. First, evacuate the pus, treat the surrounding cellulitis with antibiotics — only then consider using NPWT.
- **Necrotic tissue and eschar**. Wait with the VAC until the wound is thoroughly debrided!
- **Underlying osteomyelitis**. There is no point in using NPWT in a wound that is constantly 'fed' by the infected bone below it.
- **Exposed vital structures**. Applying the VAC system directly over exposed organs or structures can be dangerous. It can desiccate and damage exposed blood vessels (bleeding!); it can damage exposed nerves; it can fistulate exposed intestine (unless it is adequately protected). It should be used only by responsible surgical specialists who know how to protect these structures by using dedicated barriers.
- **Ischemic limbs**. The application of negative pressure to treat wounds directly due to ischemia, or to wounds developing in limbs with some degree of ischemia (e.g. diabetic feet), can further damage the wound or the susceptible periwound. Lower suction pressures (-40 to -50mmHg) are recommended. **But be careful. Talk to the vascular surgeon**. I attempted low-pressure NPWT on the forefoot amputation stump in a diabetic patient whose foot appeared well perfused. Two days later, the surrounding skin turned pale and blistered.

- **Coagulopathy and patients on anticoagulants. It is not an absolute contraindication but a plea for cautiousness.** As NPWT promotes vascularity and granulation of the wound, bleeding may develop. You don't want the patient showing up in the emergency room with the canister full of blood and blood running out the sides of the adhesive barrier.
- **Malignancy.** The use of NPWT has previously been discouraged in wounds associated with local malignancy (e.g. after resection of a sarcoma or melanoma) due to the fear that it could promote the growth of malignant cells. **Such a concept has now been abandoned.** The VAC system can be safely used in such cases, improving palliation by clearing exudate and eliminating odor.

## What do patients need to consider before receiving a wound VAC?

**Patients must realize that:**

- They will be connected to a heavy (and noisy) mobile suction apparatus, which they will have to carry around day and night.
- It may limit their activities.
- It requires them to be careful so the device does not disconnect or the dressing does not peel off the wound, thus losing suction.
- It may occasionally malfunction and require urgent intervention. Trips to the emergency room (where there may be no one skilled in NPWT) are not uncommon.
- **Consequently, in some patients (e.g. living alone, no immediate access to help, etc.), the use of VAC is not practical.**

## A few technical points

Each of you will hopefully learn from your local wound care guru the basics on how to apply NPWT, including all the various tricks. Besides, you can watch many of the available instructive videos online. **I only wish to add some technical points based on what I see in patients coming to my clinic with VAC dressings applied in 'St. Elsewhere' hospitals, clinics or nursing homes:**

- **The periwound.** The skin surrounding the wound, when directly covered by the adhesive barrier, is susceptible to damage — by direct negative pressure, exudate siphoning from the wound, and, in some cases, sensitivity to the adhesive material. Applying a protective cream or paste (e.g. a zinc-based paste or a hydrocolloid-based paste like Stomahesive®) around the wound is a good solution. **Even better is this 'trick' I often use**: I cut strips from an adhesive patch of Stomahesive® (the material incorporated along the border of colostomy bags) and place them around the periphery of the wound. It protects the periwound and adheres firmly to the adhesive barrier, helping to prevent 'air leaks' and suction loss. Adding some Stomahesive® paste to fill skin folds improves the system's airtightness.

- **Sponge management**. The porous sponge inserted into the wound, which transmits suction to its deep spaces and tunnels, is often mismanaged. **I have observed 'wound care providers' that pack the wounds with much too large pieces of foam**. **And they do it over and over again. Such tight packing prevents healing — it doesn't allow the wound to fill in, to contract. It results in what I call a 'forever VAC'**: patients returning for VAC system changes for months (!), but their wounds are not smaller (surprise...). **Instead, the sponge should be sized slightly smaller than the cavity (~0.5cm). During each change of dressings, the cavity or 'tunnel' should be measured, and yet again, a smaller sponge reinserted. Don't stuff the sponge in, but fill it loosely!** (And of course, do not lose or forget pieces of sponge in the depth of the wound. It is uncommon, but we see it from time to time, as the edges of the tailored sponge can be friable and detach, forming a foreign body that can fester.)

## What do the patients need to be aware of while they have a wound VAC?

**Patients and/or those who care for them must be knowledgeable about the mechanisms of the device**: how it is connected to the wound, how the wound is sealed to maintain negative pressure; they must fully comprehend what to do when and if the negative pressure (the suction) is lost. **It is especially crucial for patients who undergo NPWT at home!**

**If suction is lost for any reason, patients should contact their wound care provider immediately so VAC therapy can be restored.** If this is impossible (e.g. over the weekend), they should know how to REMOVE the VAC dressing from the wound, irrigate it, and dress it with a 'simple' dressing until the VAC can be restored. **This is CRUCIAL: a wound which is disconnected from the suction and still sealed is like an undrained abscess full of pus — very rapidly it can cause invasive local infection and systemic sepsis!**

**Patients must understand that for the VAC system to succeed, the wound must be clean of any necrotic dead tissue**. So, if 'dark' or foul-smelling exudate accumulates under the dressing, is seen in the tubing or canister, or if pain and fever develop, the patient should be evaluated immediately, as re-debridement and cleanup would be necessary.

## How often should the VAC system be changed?

**The prevailing recommendation is to change the dressing every 2-3 days**. For example, Monday, Wednesday, and Friday. But this schedule is not set in stone. In some wounds that are 'doing well' (e.g. granulating, decreasing drainage), I would change the VAC twice a week (e.g. Monday and Friday). **Again: features of infection, compromised dressing, and heavy drainage require more frequent changes — change as needed.**

## How long is wound VAC used for and when should you remove it?

**The simple answer is: "until it is not needed anymore" — that is, NPWT should be discontinued when the wound has reached a stage when it can heal rapidly with conventional wound care.**

**In practice, when a wound becomes flat, non-productive, clean, and granulating ('pink'), the VAC can be terminated.** From now on, the wound will heal spontaneously. (Rarely, it can be sutured or covered with a skin graft.)

## Last words

**As with any medical device — mainly when aggressively marketed by the 'industry' — NPWT is often overused or misused. More and more I see VAC devices used on 'simple' wounds — wounds which would heal rapidly with conventional measures**. It follows the dictum: "If the only tool you have is a hammer, you treat everything as if it were a nail." **Sometimes it seems to me that the younger generation is not aware that most wounds healed successfully before the era of negative pressure therapy.**

**A 'mini' NPWT system is available; I use the SNAP™ system.** Unlike the conventional VAC devices, which are connected to a heavy, bulky electrical suction apparatus, the SNAP™ device is connected to a tiny light container

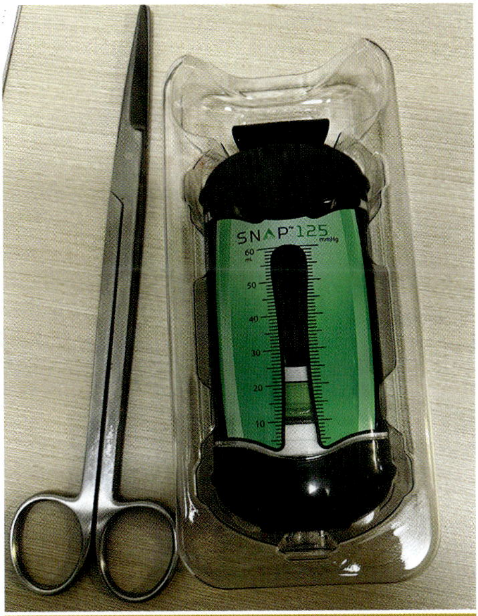


Figure 9.2. The 'mini-VAC', SNAP™.

which generates suction by mechanical, spring-activated forces. Within the tiny collecting cartridge, the exudate is converted to gel. It fits in the patient's pocket and is perfect for smaller, less productive, but deep wounds (■ Figure 9.2).

**VAC devices and their use are immensely expensive. A few weeks of use can translate to thousands of dollars!** (depending on the specific products and quantity of material used).

**"NPWT has revolutionized the treatment of complex problem wounds. However, these methods should be used selectively and knowledgeably. The indication should be correct, and one must know when enough is enough, and the VAC should be discontinued. A dedicated wound care specialist must periodically assess patients receiving NPWT to monitor progress and/or determine the need for alternative measures. Unfortunately, this is not always the case, and we see patients treated with VAC unnecessarily and 'forever' — the 'forever' VAC."**

# Chapter 10

## Palliative care

*Some wounds are never going to heal!*

**The realization that some wounds are never going to heal, and many of the wounds that heal after months of dedicated care will recur, can be frustrating to the 'newbie' in the field of wound care.** It is why the 'wound care industry' is thriving — the same patients returning again and again, until they die or decide to see a 'better' wound care specialist... but, fortunately, some do achieve long-term cure.

**Such patients require 'palliative care', not only to address pain, odor, drainage, and infection, but also dignity and even hope. These wounds usually develop due to underlying advanced diseases associated with immobility, frailty, and malnutrition — as discussed in the previous pages.**

Below are a few examples.

**An 85-year-old diabetic male who underwent forefoot (transmetatarsal) amputation.** He was hobbling around using an 'orthopedic shoe', but a year later developed a **full-thickness plantar pressure ulcer**. His foot was well perfused, but the wound resisted various prolonged local treatments. **At some point, an MRI showed features of osteomyelitis, and below-the-knee amputation was recommended.** However, the patient, who didn't want to spend the rest of his life in a wheelchair, declined the amputation. I inherited him for 'maintenance' treatment of his ulcer. **He would shuffle into my office every 3 weeks, where I would pare**

**down a thick callus (which redevelops rapidly between sessions) and 'selectively' debride the edges and base of the ulcer. The wound is washed with soap and water and dressed with honey and an absorbent bordered dressing by the patient's wife every day until the subsequent encounter**. **It has been going on for 2 years — the patient continues to walk around his house and yard (■ Figure 10.1)**.

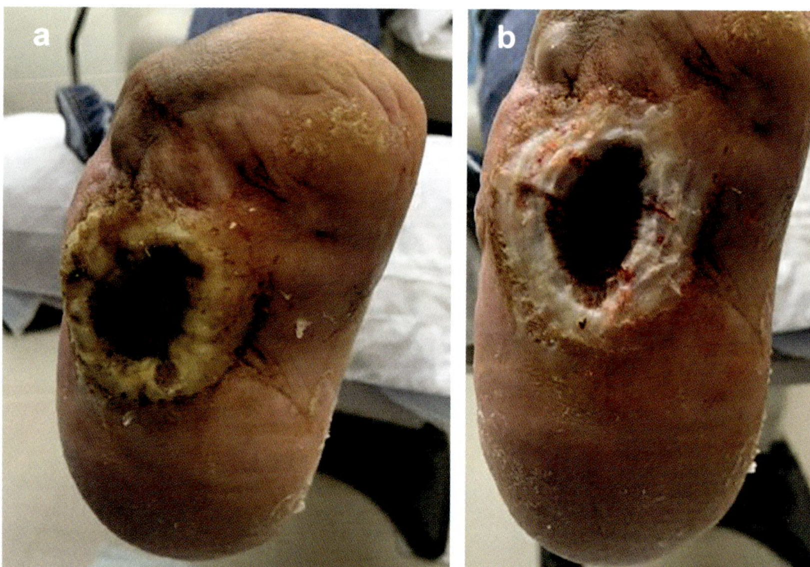


**Figure 10.1. A diabetic patient after transmetatarsal amputation. a) Note the callus developing around the wound every few weeks. b) After debridement.**

**A 45-year-old male, born with spina bifida, leading to numerous complications. He eventually ended up with a bilateral high above-knee amputation and was wheelchair-bound**. Over the years, he developed recurrent pressure ulcers on his buttocks. At the age of 49, he underwent extensive debridement of the ulcers and the underlying infected bone, followed by musculocutaneous flap reconstruction, requiring 3 months of hospitalization. **The ulcers recurred promptly**. He presented to my clinic with foul-smelling, necrotic, infected ulcers (■ Figure 10.2a). Cultures from the underlying exposed bone grew *Staphylococcus aureus*. After receiving a diverting colostomy I debrided him in the operating room (■ Figure 10.2b) and started local care with honey. **The poor guy**

**refused any further major reconstructive procedures, so I discharged him with local care: daily showers, honey onto the wound, strips of absorptive Aquacel® into the deep recesses, covered with Mepilex®, and long-term oral doxycycline. He continued to cruise on his wheelchair across town — comfortable, his wound contracted (■ Figure 10.2c), not smelly, dry, and pain-free.** Over the next few years, I would see him periodically in the clinic until he succumbed to a massive myocardial infarction (he smoked two packs a day supplemented with marijuana).

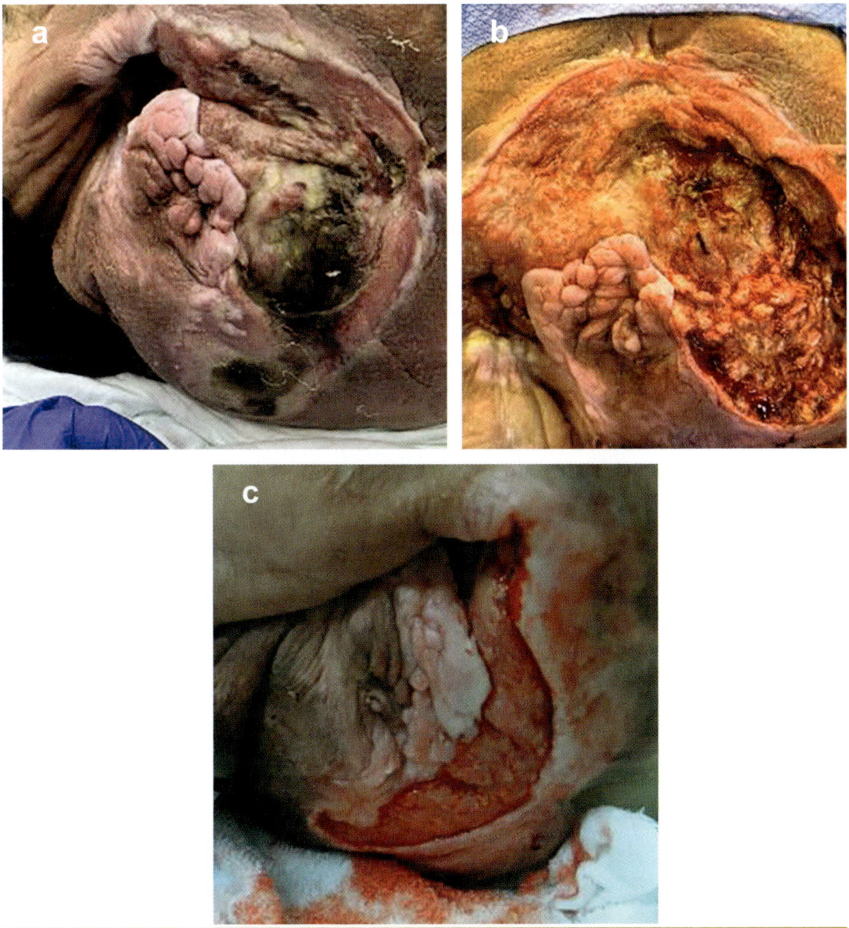

Figure 10.2. A bilateral above-knee amputee with a non-healable pressure ulcer of his buttocks. a) Before surgical debridement. b) A few days after debridement. c) Six months later, with 'maintenance treatment'.

**A 61-year-old man, previously a drug addict and alcoholic, a heavy smoker with oxygen-dependent COPD, who developed stasis dermatitis and lipodermatosclerosis of his lower limbs.** He would be repeatedly admitted with bacterial cellulitis associated with swollen, ulcerated, weepy legs; there were numerous attempts to fit him with various compression garments that he wouldn't or couldn't apply properly (■ Figure 10.3). **Finally, we tried the Unna boots. It worked perfectly. We see him every 3 or 4 weeks (whenever he finds a neighbor who can drive him in), remove the Unna boots, clean and brush his legs and feet to remove reaccumulating desquamated tissue (typical for this condition), and reapply the Unna boots. It is how we have been 'maintaining' him now for 3 years: he is happy schlepping himself around the house in his Unna boots — his legs are not swollen, not weepy, and there have been no further episodes of cellulitis.**

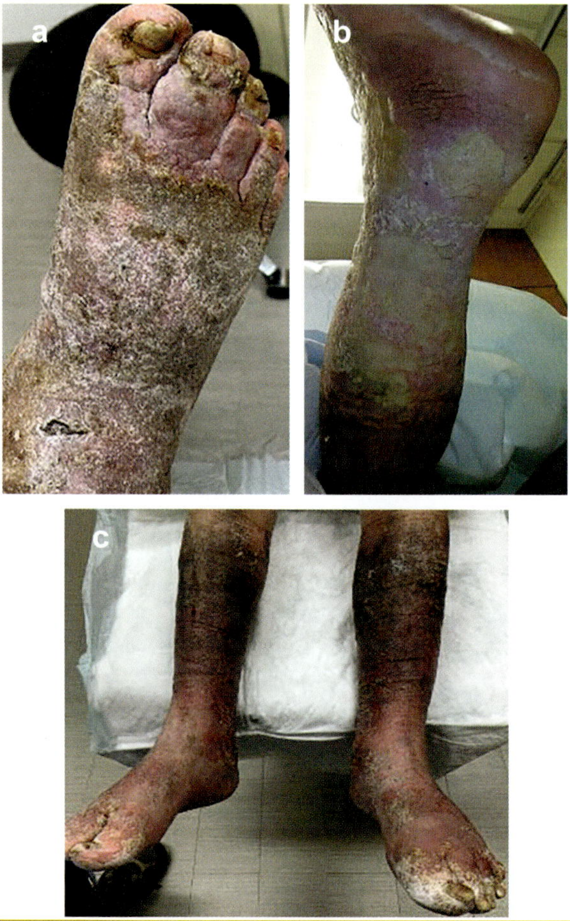


**Figure 10.3. a) and b) Intractable stasis dermatitis/lipodermatosclerosis. c) Six months later, the skin is now healed, with no swelling or recurrent infection.**

Of course, there are many other examples: like the terminal cancer patient with a giant bedsore or the stage 4 melanoma patient with a fungating tumor in his groin. **They all deserve to cruise towards the end with dignity and relative comfort**. You should treat them as 'conservatively' as possible along the lines described in this book: limited debridement in the office (if possible), and management of infection and moisture control. **Odor is a significant concern**. One of the primary sources of odor are the anaerobic bacteria multiplying in these wounds. Dressings impregnated with silver or charcoal, or topical metronidazole, are helpful. **But I find that applying a generous dose of honey to the wound is most effective**.

**"Palliative wound care: comfort before cure and less is more."**

# Chapter 11

## Prevention

A timeless aphorism:
*An ounce of prevention is worth more than a million pounds of cure.*
A cliché? Yes. But true!

**By now, after reading the previous chapters, you surely know why wounds develop, what are the factors that make people susceptible to them, and how to control those factors — namely, how to prevent the wounds from forming or recurring. But it is easier said than done! The blame rests on both of us — us in the 'medical industry' and the patients themselves.**

### The 'medical industry'

Detailed protocols for preventing the various pressure injuries ('pressure sores') are widely available in books and online, taught in nursing teaching programs, and implemented in hospitals and nursing homes. They include:

- Initial and periodic risk assessment.
- Frequent repositioning.
- Daily skin inspection, focusing on high-risk areas.
- Use of pressure-reducing equipment (e.g. specialized mattresses, cushions).

- Regular skin care to avoid prolonged soiling and excessive moisture.
- Adequate nutrition.

**Yes, each nurse and nurse manager knows all the above, but pressure wounds still develop. Why?** The nurse managers run around in their high heels, lead Zoom meetings, and write protocols. The nurses are constantly documenting on their laptops (including recording that all measures to prevent skin injury have been met), and the nursing aids — the ones who actually come into physical contact with the patients — are overwhelmed. And the doctors (i.e. 'providers' these days)? They, hospitalists, specialists, whatever, are running around trying to solve the acute problem (ASAP, until the insurance runs out) and meeting their productivity requirements. It is an 'industry', remember? **In my experience, such a scenario is much more common in large hospitals than in your little community or rural establishment**.

So, you spend 3 months curing a deep pressure sore on the buttocks. Then the patient develops respiratory distress and is shipped to a top-rated ivory tower in the city, only to return to you after 2 weeks with the original pressure ulcer recurring plus a fresh pressure ulcer on the heel.

## Patients and their families

They are often responsible as well. **Poor compliance with preventive measures is a huge problem**. The 'big boy', whose huge venous ulcer you managed to heal after 5 months, decides not to wear his compression garments during a Caribbean cruise or a hunting expedition, and returns to you with a recurrence. And so, it goes on.

**But in many cases, it's hard to blame the patients**. They are old and frail, often with declining cognitive abilities. Some are lonely, with no immediate human support — no one to help them reapply the compression stocking or the heel protector, or to tell them not to sit all day in the wheelchair. And then come the **financial issues: chronic wounds are much more common in the indigent population**. When the old Ford truck breaks down, or the social security money runs out at the end of the month, one has to postpone the visit to the clinic and subsist on the 'healthy diet' of 'mac and cheese'. However, occasionally one sees one of these patients with a new iPhone in his hand and a pack of Marlboro sticking out of his front pocket...

**All of this is obvious. But instead of the 'blame game', let us see what we, the wound care specialists, can do to improve the situation in the individual patient.**

**During each encounter, we need to dedicate a few minutes to educating (and re-educating) the patient and his family or caregivers on how to prevent the wound from recurring and new wounds from developing.** The factors listed in ■ Table 3.2 in ➲ Chapter 3 should be used selectively for each patient. For example:

- Do you still smoke? Stop or cut down!
- What do you eat? Enough proteins and vitamins?
- Are you taking your diuretics?
- Is your diabetes controlled?
- Are you elevating your legs when resting?
- Are you wearing the compression stockings properly?
- Are your heels protected when lying down?
- Is your wheelchair well-padded?
- Are you changing positions frequently when lying down or sitting?

**It is our responsibility to communicate regularly with home wound care teams and nursing homes** to instruct them on exactly what you want them to do. We must be in direct contact with the patients' primary care docs or internists to inform them of findings that require their intervention (e.g. worsening congestive heart failure). We are responsible for seeing that the patient receives the correct orthotic devices from the medical supply shops.

**In sum: our approach must be 'holistic'**. Yes, the vascular surgeon focuses on the occluded artery, the cardiologist on the coronary stent, the endocrinologist on the HbA1c, the general surgeon on the tumor he removes from the groin. **Still, you — the wound care specialist — you must focus on the whole patient!**

**"Add in your mind a 'P' to the TIME acronym for prevention — P-TIME! And don't forget the C for compression."**

# Chapter 12

## Gimmicks

*Try to avoid gimmicks and fads — use proven remedies!*

Some readers, especially 'established' wound care specialists, would probably object to the use of the term 'gimmick' ('a trick or device intended to attract attention, publicity, or business') in the context of wound care. Instead, they would prefer this chapter to be titled 'innovative wound care products'. But I favor the term 'gimmick' for the reasons outlined below...

You may have heard about or encountered some of the 'innovative wound care products' — offered by enthusiastic company reps visiting your clinic who hand out shiny brochures, or used by equally enthusiastic (or gullible) colleagues. **Here are a few examples**: bioengineered tissue and cellular products (e.g. bioengineered skin graft), 'smart' wound dressings (with biosensors to monitor wound conditions in real time), injectable hydrogels, various growth factors (delivered into the wound), AI and digital wound assessment, placenta-based products (there are 28 different placenta-based skin substitute products available in the USA), and so forth — the list is long.

**The common denominator of all such products is that the evidence supporting their advantage over 'conventional' treatment is flimsy at best, and that they are immensely costly**. In previous chapters, I repeatedly pointed to the poor quality of evidence deriving from 'wound care studies': industry-supported studies, mostly published in obscure journals — gathered from many 'unknown' centers, questionable randomization, and 'suspicious' meta-analyses (i.e. gathering results from many faulty studies into a meta-analysis doesn't make it more credible). **The same applies to these 'innovative' treatments.**

**Using ultra-expensive products of questionable value also raises ethical issues. For example**:

There are numerous **placenta-derived wound care products on the market. Here I cite from an article in *The New York Times* (April 10, 2025) entitled, "Medicare bleeds billions on pricey bandages, and doctors get a cut"**: "Made of dried bits of placenta, the paper-thin patches cover stubborn wounds and can cost thousands per square inch ($5,948)... In the past few years, dozens of unstudied and costly products flooded the market... Some doctors buy the products at large discounts but charge Medicare the full sticker price, pocketing the difference. Spending on skin substitutes exceeded $10 billion in 2024, more than double the figure in 2023. Medicare now spends more on bandages than on ambulance rides, anesthesia, and CT scans... In one patient in Nevada, Medicare spent $14 million on skin substitutes over the course of a year..."

**Another example: injectable hydrogels are promoted as advantageous for deep-tunneling wounds**. Again, the evidence is flimsy, but what about the cost? The current price of a single injection ranges from the upper hundreds to over a thousand dollars. Now compare it to the cost of a dose of honey and some straightforward dressings.

**Fortunately, it seems that such 'innovative wound therapies' find it hard to penetrate routine clinical practice**. There are a few reasons:

- Most insurance companies do not cover the product, so it is unaffordable for clinics and patients (unless companies find loopholes, e.g. as *The New York Times* article mentioned above).
- The regulatory bodies do not approve the product because of a lack of 'evidence' and the need for specialized infrastructure, equipment, and coordination.
- Most providers are not 'suckers' — **they are reluctant to depart from established, familiar products in favor of some gimmicks**.

**I hope you are not a sucker, either. Not one of those who rushes to place yet another thousand-dollar piece of thin 'bio-dressing' on a non-healable wound!**

## Hyperbaric oxygen therapy (HBOT) for wound treatment

**I choose to mention HBOT at the end of this chapter; even it cannot be described as 'innovative' or a 'gimmick'.** It is not 'innovative' because it was introduced into wound care in Japan around 50 years ago. It is most probably not a 'gimmick' because some studies suggest that HBOT combined with 'standard wound care' improves the healing rate of chronic wounds, especially in **diabetic foot ulcers, where it helps avoid amputation.** However, such an opinion is not absolute, as **HBOT studies are, yet again, of suboptimal quality; thus, the topic has been clouded in controversy since I graduated from medical school in 1979...**

### Why is HBOT not widely used for chronic wounds?

There are a few reasons:

- **Availability**: there are a few hyperbaric oxygen therapy centers, especially in major cities, and the chamber capacity is limited. (In the USA, only around 1000 centers are offering HBOT; a typical session lasts 90-120 minutes.)
- **High cost**: each session costs a few hundred dollars; a typical course requires numerous sessions with a total cost above 10,000 dollars. (Insurance coverage is variable and usually restricted to diabetic foot ulcers with a risk of amputation.)
- **Potential complications**: they are relatively rare, but the risk increases with more sessions; for example: middle ear and sinus barotrauma, ocular effects, oxygen toxicity causing seizures, and pneumothorax.

**Now you can see why HBOT is rarely used**: is it practical to send an elderly diabetic patient with a chronic ulcer to the nearest HBOT center (in my case, it's 2 hours away) for 40-60 sessions of HBOT? It is not practical for me or most of you. However, if you practice in an urban environment near an HBOT center, you can try it out. This way, you will support this lucrative business.

## Electrical stimulation

Electrical stimulation has been promoted as a valuable adjunct to wound care through various mechanisms. Physical or occupational therapists use transcutaneous electrical nerve stimulation for multiple pain syndromes and neuromuscular indications, so it is no wonder these specialties are the primary users of this method for wound care. However, the evidence to support the use of electrical stimulation is far from being perfect, and it has never been adopted into the 'mainstream' of wound care in the USA or around the world. **It appears to be yet another 'voodoo' office practice to lure gullible wound bearers**.

**"According to Dr. Marcia Angell, the pharmaceutical industry is 'now primarily a marketing machine to sell drugs of dubious benefit'. This obviously includes many of the 'novel' wound care products."**

# PART III

## Specific wounds

In this section, I will discuss in some detail the various types of wounds introduced in ➲ Chapter 2 and listed in ■ Table 2.1. By now, you are familiar with the basics of wound management; let us be more specific and see how those basics apply to wounds across various etiologies. Please study Parts I and II of the book, and consult them as you read Part III.

Most such entities deserve a separate book. And indeed, entire books are available to cover topics such as 'The diabetic foot'. **But here I will simplify things — focusing on what you, the humble 'wound care provider', must know to treat the wound. For example, I will discuss how to treat the diabetic ulcer but not how to amputate the necrotic toe**.

Of course, some repetitions are intentional and unavoidable.

# Chapter 13

## Venous ulcers

*Walk — don't stand. Elevate (the legs) — don't sit. And above all — compress (the legs).*

**Venous ulcers (some call them 'varicose' ulcers) develop in the legs of patients suffering from long-term venous hypertension.**

### Pathophysiology

**In the 'pure' form, they develop in patients with varicose veins**: the incompetent valves within the veins cause pooling of blood around the ankle region, increasing venous pressure, which is transmitted to the skin and rendering it ischemic. Initially, the affected skin exhibits features of **stasis dermatitis**; eventually, after years, an ulcer develops.

**The varicose veins can be of two types**:

- **Primary varicose veins**: affecting only the *superficial veins* (the greater or lesser saphenous vein systems). They typically develop in younger, healthier patients with a genetic predisposition; they are more common in women.
- **Secondary varicose veins**: when the venous hypertension results from occlusion of the *deep venous system*, usually due to previous episodes of deep vein thrombosis (DVT). Other causes of damage to the deep veins include previous trauma, tumors, etc.

**As I mentioned previously, many of the so-called 'varicose ulcers' we see today are not 'pure'. They are of 'mixed' etiology — the most common**

**being morbid obesity leading to both elevated venous and lymphatic hypertension.** In such cases, varicose veins are often absent, and so better terms to use are 'stasis dermatitis' and 'stasis ulcer' (see also ➲ Chapter 19). **Below, we will deal with the 'pure' form.**

## Clinical features

**Findings on examination are characteristic:**

- **Varicose veins are present:** above and below the knee in the distribution of the greater saphenous vein, and below the knee and posteriorly in the distribution of the lesser saphenous vein. **To see the varicosities, you must examine the patient in the standing position!**
- **The ulcers:** of variable size, are shallow with well-demarcated edges. They may be red or covered with yellowish exudate. In some cases, they may be weeping — particularly if associated with significant leg edema or superimposed cellulitis. **Typically, the ulcers develop along the distal course of the greater saphenous vein on the distal-medial area of the leg (above the medial malleolus).** But atypical locations (e.g. higher up on the shin) are common, especially in the 'mixed etiology' variants. **The ulcers are tender and painful. The pain increases when the legs are dependent during the day and is relieved with elevation. Note that with ischemic ulcers, the situation is reversed:** symptoms improve when the legs are dependent and increase during the night. **Diabetic ulcers, on the other hand, are commonly painless due to the underlying peripheral neuropathy.**
- **Surrounding skin:** is *invariably* affected with chronic changes of 'stasis dermatitis' and lipodermatosclerosis, the intensity of which depends on the chronicity of the condition. The skin is reddish, brown, and tense: 'brownish induration'.
- **Leg edema:** it is much more common and pronounced in patients with secondary varicose veins, but it is often present in longstanding primary varicosities as well.
- **Legs affected by longstanding stasis dermatitis are susceptible to bacterial cellulitis.** It causes a sudden increase in swelling, with the legs becoming red and tender; new 'weeping' ulcers develop or recur.

## Diagnosis and investigations

**Clinical diagnosis is straightforward based on the features listed above.** Many of these patients report a previous history of similar ulcers, and they know already how they will be treated; some understand why they have recurred — non-compliance with proper compression.

**In some cases, further investigations are necessary**:

- **Duplex ultrasound**: in patients with significant leg edema and/or 'minimal' varicosities, I would order this test to exclude acute or longstanding thrombosis in the deep venous system.
- **ABI**: in patients with unpalpable peripheral pulses, I want to rule out an ischemic component that is contributing to the ulcer and would prevent healing.

## Treatment

**The treatment of venous ulcers is clear-cut and ages-old: when the venous hypertension is controlled, the ulcer will heal**. Already in the 5th century BC, Hippocrates understood that leg elevation and compression would heal these ulcers. In the 1990s, when I worked in South Africa, we would confine these patients to bed, with elevated legs for a few weeks (!) and invariably even huge venous healed. **Obviously, such a regimen is unimaginable these days — the current mainstay of treatment is compression**.

**So, treat the ulcer, treat the associated cellulitis (if present), and compress the leg, along the lines outlined in ➲ Chapter 8, and the ulcer will heal**. As you know by now, there are many ways to treat the ulcer and various compression methods. **In my hands, a minor debridement, some honey, and an Unna boot are an optimal combination**.

**Treatment of associated cellulitis**: the causative bacteria are mostly *Staphylococcus aureus* and *Streptococcus pyogenes* (Group A). Both are susceptible to **cephalexin**, which is my drug of choice for empirical treatment of leg cellulitis. In the 'mild' cases (i.e. no systemic features of infection), I treat the affected area with one of the agents described in ➲ Chapter 6, place one of the dressings described in ➲ Chapter 7, apply compression (➲ Chapter 8), and prescribe the antibiotic for 7-10 days. **When systemic repercussions of the infection are present, the patient should be admitted** for a course of i.v. antibiotics (e.g. cefazolin or amoxicillin-clavulanate).

**How fast should the ulcer diminish in size?** The range is 0.5-1.4cm per week, with a 30-50% reduction in size after a month. After 3-5 months, most ulcers should heal (■ Figure 13.1).

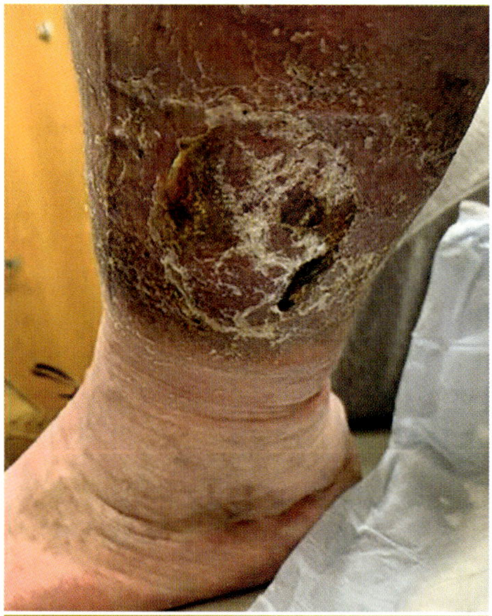

**Figure 13.1. Large recurrent venous ulcer in an obese patient almost healed after 3 months of treatment with an Unna boot. Note the extensive 'stasis dermatitis' in the background.**

## Surgical options

There are a few surgical options:

- **Varicose vein ablation: primary varicose veins are potentially curable by surgical intervention, which, by eliminating venous hypertension, prevents ulcer recurrence**. In the 'old days', I would 'strip' out the incompetent saphenous vein system. However, **currently, minimally invasive endovascular procedures** — ambulatory, performed under local anesthesia, avoiding large wounds — which ablate veins with energy applied from within, are taking over in most places. **Therefore, after the ulcer has healed, I would refer such patients (those who are relatively 'young and fit') to a vascular or general surgeon qualified in venous endovascular ablation procedures**. **Of course, ablating the superficial venous system in patients with secondary varicose veins (where the deep system is occluded) is contraindicated**.

- **Skin grafting**. Covering the ulcers with partial-thickness skin grafts is considered a 'second-line' option reserved for very large ulcers (>25cm$^2$) that fail to heal after prolonged conservative treatment (e.g. ~6 months). **To be successful, the bed of the ulcer has to be 'clean' (e.g. healthy granulation tissue) and, above all, the underlying cause of the ulcer — the venous hypertension — has to be well controlled; otherwise, skin grafting would be a futile exercise!** Results are 'mixed'. I never had to resort to this option.

**An additional management option is the drug pentoxifylline**, which the literature has advocated as a proven adjunct in the management of venous ulcers. It is claimed that it accelerates healing by improving microcirculatory flow and modulating inflammation. Despite being recommended by various 'guidelines' and 'societies', this relatively cheap drug is rarely used for this indication in the USA. I don't know why… but I never used it.

## How to prevent recurrence

**Some studies report a recurrence rate of over 50% within a year, and as high as 80% after several years of follow-up**. Overall (patterns of practice vary from location to location), less than a third of patients with healed varicose ulcers are referred for vein ablation procedures. **So, how do you prevent recurrence in most cases?**

- **Lifestyle change**: walk more, sit less, elevate legs when resting, and lose weight (easier said than done!).
- **Lifelong compression. It is the key! With inadequate or inconsistent compression** (patients will always find some excuses: "it's too hot… too tight… I forgot to take it with me on vacation…"), **the ulcer will surely recur**.
- **How high should the compression pressure be?** According to the various guidelines, patients need compression of 30-40mmHg to prevent recurrence. Such garments at these pressure levels are considered '*extra-firm*' and require a prescription to be covered by insurance and to be correctly fitted by a certified seller. However, at least half of the patients cannot tolerate such pressures, or are unable to don the '*extra-firm*' garments. **So, to improve compliance, I often compromise and recommend 20-30mmHg — '*firm*' — garments**. These are available over the counter. There are many options (see ➲ Chapter 8).

**"There is no need to reinvent the wheel. Our ancestors knew it many thousands ago: elevation and compression prevent and cure all venous ulcers."**

# Chapter 14

## Diabetic ulcers

*The treatment of 'diabetic feet' doesn't end when the ulcer is healed or the toe or feet have been amputated. The ulcer must be prevented and treated, continuously, as long as the patient lives!*

**The American obesity pandemic (now spreading around the world) produces a large number of type 2 diabetic patients. Approximately 2% of such patients will develop diabetic foot ulcers (DFUs)** each year; the lifetime risk of DFU in each patient is ~20-30%. These figures translate to the astounding number of 1.5-2 million annual new cases of DFUs ('diabetic feet'). No wonder that DFUs and their complications are a leading cause of admissions and amputations in diabetic patients.

**The care of 'diabetic feet' falls under many specialties**: podiatry, vascular surgery, general surgery, infectious diseases, endocrinology, and others. **What is your role — the role of the wound care specialist?**

**Your role is to assess the patient referred to you with a DFU and decide**:

- Can I continue with standard wound care and expect healing?
- Must I refer the patient to one of the surgical specialists for surgical debridement or amputation?
- Should I refer him to vascular surgery for revascularization?

Another role would be to continue treating the wounds after the surgeons have completed their job... and know when to send them back to the surgeons — which, unfortunately, is required so often.

## Pathophysiology

I already mentioned (➲ Chapter 2) why diabetic patients are prone to 'diabetic feet'. But let us dwell on this a little deeper.

**The pathophysiologic triad responsible for DFUs comprises:**

1. **Diabetic neuropathy.**
2. **Peripheral vascular disease.**
3. **Metabolic dysfunction and immune deficiency.**

Here are a few details:

- **Peripheral neuropathy is the key factor** (many of such patients have adequate arterial perfusion to their feet, and their blood sugars are well controlled, but still, they develop ulcers!). **The neuropathy, in turn, includes another triad**:
  - **motor neuropathy**: it weakens the foot muscles, resulting in deformities that produce plantar areas subject to pressure injuries;
  - **sensory neuropathy**: the patient loses 'protective' sensation in his foot and toes and does not appreciate any minor injuries from pressure or external trauma (e.g. ill-fitting shoes, scalding water);
  - **autonomic neuropathy**: impaired sweat production leads to dry skin, which is prone to the development of fissures and breakdown.
- **Peripheral vascular disease**: small- and/or medium-sized artery disease is commonly present in diabetic patients. When significant, it contributes to the formation of DFUs and prevents their healing.
- **Metabolic dysfunction and immune deficiency**: hyperglycemia due to poor diabetes control impairs wound healing and weakens local immune mechanisms, exposing ulcers to infection.

## Clinical features

**DFUs develop on the weight-bearing surfaces** — plantar bony prominences such as the heads of the metatarsal bones. **They can also develop on the toes** — on the base of the toes, burdened by constant weight, or on the dorsal aspect of the toes rubbing against the shoes (hammertoes are a risk factor).

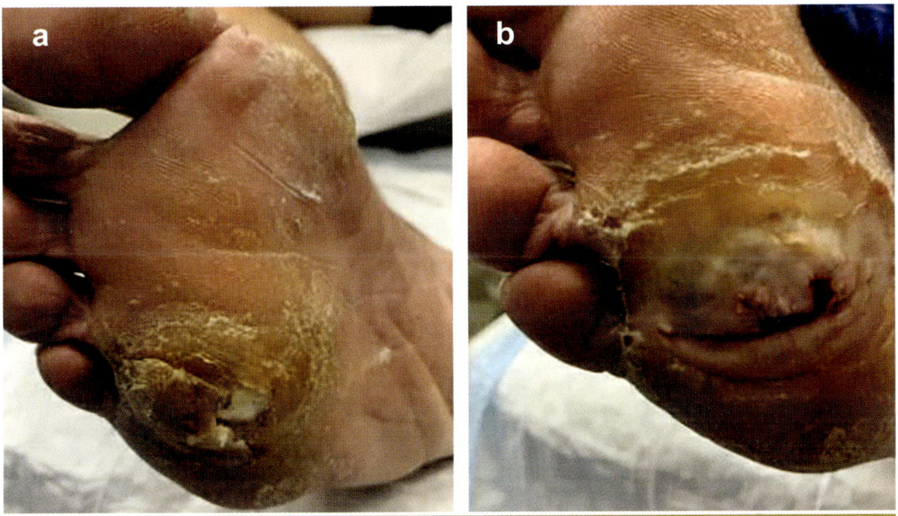


**Figure 14.1. A DFU corresponding to the head of the 5th metatarsal. a) The callus overlying the ulcer. b) The ulcer visible after paring down the callus.**

**Overlying and surrounding calluses are a characteristic finding. Often, the ulcer is hidden under the callus; it is only when the callus is pared down the full extent of the ulcer that it is disclosed** (■ Figure 14.1). The ulcer typically has a crater-like appearance and is painless (remember the neuropathy). Various amounts of slough or necrotic tissue may occupy the ulcer's bed, and features of infection or ischemia can be observed in the vicinity. The finding of a swollen, red toe suggests bone involvement. In late-presenting cases, gangrene of the toe or foot could have already set in.

**Assessing the depth of the ulcer and what structures are exposed is a crucial first step in your decision-making**. The literature offers various grading or classification systems of DFUs. But as always, the more grading systems exist, the more confusing they become, and the less likely they are used by clinicians — including myself. **I prefer describing what I see**:

- **Is the ulcer 'superficial'**, not penetrating the skin (partial thickness)?
- **Is the ulcer deep**, when the subcutaneous fat (the pulp space) is exposed (full thickness)?
- **Are there any deep structures (tendons, joint capsule, bone) visible or palpable?**

**Inserting a sterile metal probe** (you can use sterile small artery forceps) into the depth of the ulcer is an important step: **when and if the probe**

**touches the underlying bone — a positive 'probe-to-bone' test — is highly suggestive (but not diagnostic) of underlying osteomyelitis.**

**Of course, you should carefully assess the whole limb beyond the confines of the ulcer: is there any spreading cellulitis beyond the confines of the ulcer?**

## Investigations

- **X-ray of the foot.** Many of these patients will have already had one; if not, I would obtain one routinely. Beyond the typical findings expected in the 'diabetic foot' — osteopenia, bone and joint deformities and subluxations ('Charcot foot') — **I look for features of soft-tissue infection (gas pockets) or osteomyelitis (cortical destruction).** If such features are absent, the **initial X-ray serves as a baseline**, as radiographic changes of osteomyelitis can be delayed by weeks or months; therefore, one must compare the fresh X-ray to previous ones, if available.
- **MRI. MRI is the 'gold standard' for diagnosing 'diabetic foot' complications — bone destruction and soft-tissue infection.** It also accurately delineates the magnitude of the neuroarthropathy. **So, when the X-ray is 'non-conclusive' (as it often is) and/or I suspect bone or deep-space involvement (e.g. positive 'probe-to-bone test' test), I would order an MRI.**
- **TBI (Toe-Brachial Index). I order this test routinely as a baseline.** As I mentioned in ➲ Chapter 4, ABI measurements are not accurate in diabetic patients because their leg arteries are non-compressible due to severe calcification, leading to falsely high ABI readings (ABI of 1.3 or higher). For the same reason, even palpable foot pulses may not exclude ischemia. However, the small toe arteries are spared and provide 'true' arterial pressure. Toe pressures are now routinely measured during ABI tests, providing essential information. **In general, a toe pressure below 50mmHg in a diabetic patient is considered pathological. A pressure below 30mmHg suggests severe ischemia and a very low likelihood of spontaneous wound healing, or the healing of any foot amputation wound.**
- **Wound cultures.** As discussed in ➲ Chapter 4, all chronic wounds are colonized with bacteria. **Thus, DFUs should not be routinely cultured unless there are clinical signs and symptoms of infection. The bacteriology of DFUs is polymicrobial. Gram-positive cocci** (e.g. *Staphylococcus aureus*, MRSA, *Streptococcus*

species, *Enterococcus* species) are the most common initial pathogens, especially in mild-to-moderate, community-acquired infections. **Gram-negative aerobic rods** (e.g. *Pseudomonas aeruginosa*, *Escherichia coli*, *Klebsiella* species, *Proteus* species) tend to appear in more chronic, severe, or hospital-acquired infections. **Anaerobic bacteria** (e.g. *Bacteroides* species, *Clostridium* species) are typically found in deeper, or necrotic wounds.

## Treatment

**So now that you have assessed the patient, you need to decide whether you can keep treating this patient in your wound care clinic or if you need to ask your surgical colleagues for help.**

### When to refer out?

- **Features of invasive-spreading infection** (pus pouring from the wound, spreading cellulitis, gas in the soft tissues) **indicate an *emergency*. The patient needs i.v. antibiotics and aggressive surgical debridement. Call your podiatrist or general surgeon.**
- **Visible tissue gangrene. Cases of 'wet' gangrene** (the dead tissue is 'productive', inflamed, and infected) **represent an *emergency*, in need of immediate surgical treatment. 'Dry' gangrene** — shriveled, dry black eschar covering the wound — can be treated conservatively unless it becomes 'wet' (see ➲ Chapter 15).
- **Visible or palpable, exposed deep structures** (bone, tendons, joint) or a positive 'probe-to-bone' test **require an *urgent* referral to the podiatrist or surgeon.**
- **Acute critical foot ischemi**a (e.g. the whole foot and/or distal leg is blue) **requires an *emergency* referral to vascular surgery.**
- **Chronic foot ischemia.** When toe pressure is below 50mmHg, I request a ***semi-urgent* consult** with vascular surgery, considering revascularization. When toe pressure is below 30mmHg, I ask for an ***urgent*** consultation.
- **Additional imaging before referral.** The podiatrist or surgeon may want to obtain an **MRI** to serve as a road map during the surgical debridement/amputation. The vascular surgeon will likely require **CT angiography** to determine whether revascularization is a viable option. I often order these tests before sending them away. But it depends on your local circumstances.

## Management at your wound care clinic

Say you are confronted with a DFU without any of the features that require referral out, or with a patient who has already undergone surgical debridement, amputation or revascularization, and sent back to you to continue local care (including the open amputation wound of the toe or forefoot) — how to treat the patient?

**Before looking at what's specific to the 'diabetic foot', let us not forget the basics**. DFUs are treated according to the same principles outlined in ➲ Part II: remember TIME? (Tissue debridement, Infection control, Moisture balance, Edges advancement). And don't forget **compression** (the compression pressure calibrated to the estimated arterial perfusion) if leg edema is present. **Obviously, glycemic control is crucial — the higher the blood glucose and HbA1c, the less likely the wound is to heal**.

**What's specific to the 'diabetic foot'?**

**Offloading the foot. This is a keystone of management aimed at reducing pressure on the ulcerated area to allow healing**. A wide range of offloading methods exists, to be selected for each patient based on the location of the wound, the presence of infection, the patient's mobility, and his preferences. An exhaustive discussion of the various offloading methods would be beyond the scope of this little book, but here are a few basics:

- **Non-removable knee-high devices**, such as total contact casts (TCCs) or non-removable knee-high walkers, are considered the most efficient for offloading (because patients cannot remove them). However, these devices are cumbersome, causing discomfort, poor mobility — patients hate them — and are thus not commonly used.
- **Removable knee-high devices**: these are better tolerated but still cumbersome. It's impossible to drive while wearing such a device.
- **Removable ankle-high devices: can be custom-made orthopedic shoes or 'bandage' shoes**. Another example is the padded Rooke® boot, which offloads the heel and protects the forefoot.
- **Felted foam and other padding** inserted into the shoes. These can be custom-cut to target pressure points. 'Windows' can be cut out to accommodate the dressed wounds.
- **Half, 'wedge' shoes**: restrict weight bearing either to the forefoot or heel, depending on the location of the pressure point. Also called a 'post-op shoe'.
- **Non-device offloading**: scooters, crutches, wheelchairs, bed rest.

As with compression devices, the choice is vast, and selection for the individual patient is complex. You have to become familiar with what is offered by the medical supply (DME-durable medical equipment) stores in your area. A large selection of such devices is available online, but they can be expensive when purchased out of pocket. **You must advise patients what device to buy**.

And there is nothing wrong with a 'homemade' method: **I often use a 'football dressing'** to offload some feet, especially for a heel DFU (also used for a pressure heel ulcer in non-diabetics). I wrap around the foot (including the ankle) 4-5 layers of cast padding; then wrap again with a gauze bandage and an adhesive elastic bandage (Coban™ or Ace™ wrap) — until the foot looks like a bulky football. Cheap, effective, and can be replaced at home.

**Paring down the calluses**. During each encounter, continue paring down any residual calluses that may persist or reform despite offloading. The ulcer won't heal when a callus surrounds its edges. **The skin edges should be thin and flat to allow epidermal migration**. I use for this purpose a combination of a #10 blade, a disposable curette, and the Dremel® tool.

**Negative pressure wound therapy (NPWT) is of great value in selected wounds in diabetic patients — especially the non-healing feet and leg stumps of amputees (➲ Chapter 9). However, as I already mentioned, applying negative pressure on marginally perfused areas can be deleterious (■ Figure 14.2). Use it cautiously**.

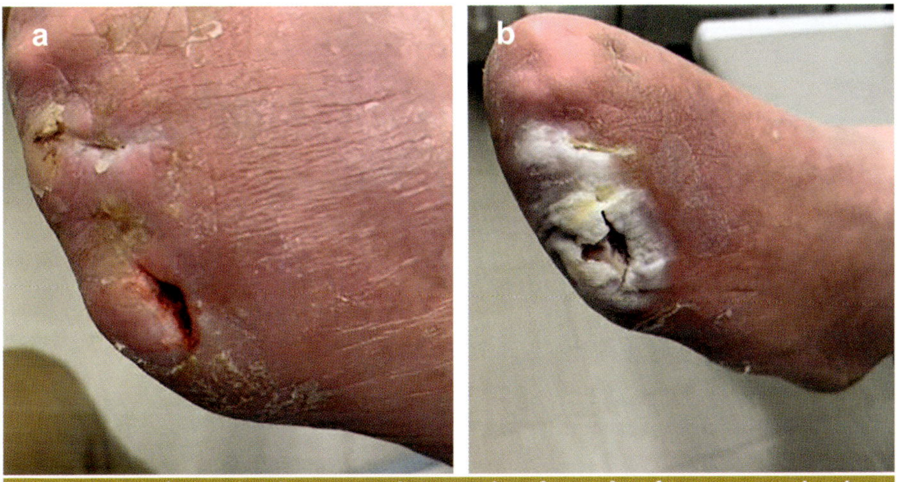


Figure 14.2. a) Non-healing wound 2 months after a forefoot amputation in a diabetic patient. b) Five days after NPWT — note the injury to the periwound.

## Operations to eliminate pressure points

**When offloading fails** (think of the diabetic office manager who continues to wear high heels to work), or **when pressure points and DFUs recur**, there are surgical options, such as bone shaving or removal, correcting deformities like bunions or hammertoes, and removing prominent or bone fragments. **It falls under the podiatrist's or orthopedic surgeon's domain**.

## Rate of healing

According to the literature, around a third of diabetic foot ulcers are expected to heal within 3 months of treatment. A 50% reduction in ulcer size after 1 month of therapy predicts healing by 3 months. About a third of DFUs never fully heal: the fate of such patients is to undergo an amputation, or (in some cases) to continue palliative 'maintenance' care (➲ Chapter 10).

## Prevention

**The recurrence rate for diabetic foot ulcers is very high**. At least half of the patients will return with a recurrence or a new DFU within a few years. Thus, a healed diabetic ulcer should not be considered a 'permanent cure' but a 'remission'. **It is our job to try to prolong such 'remissions' for as long as possible. We must educate the patient and guide them on how to avoid recurrence**:

- **Avoid minor injuries**: don't walk around barefoot. Don't immerse your feet in hot water or place them near the stove. Seek immediate medical attention for even the most trivial injury.
- **Daily self-examination**: ask for help (sometimes wives can be helpful) or use a mirror to inspect the plantar areas and the base of the toes.
- **Maintain optimal hygiene**: wash the feet in lukewarm water with mild soap, including the web spaces.
- **Avoid dry skin**: dry skin is prone to cracking, which can progress to ulcers. Hence, apply a moisturizing lotion or cream to the entire foot, but avoid the spaces between the toes.
- **Look after your nails**: trim the nails straight across with a nail clipper. Be careful not to injure the nail bed or cuticles.
- **Use proper footwear**: wear well-fitting 'offloading' and 'protective' shoes at all times, even at home. Use soft, moisture-wicking socks and change them daily. Commercial diabetic socks are available: they are non-constricting, seamless to avoid friction, provide extra padding, and are absorbent.

- **Manage 'basic' risk factors**: try to optimize your diabetes control, eat healthy food, lose weight, and stop smoking.

**I routinely refer these patients to our 'diabetes foot nurse' for periodic foot care, which includes nail care and paring of re-emerging calluses.** In the USA, Medicare and other insurance companies cover a 'foot exam and treatment' every 6 months for diabetic patients with peripheral neuropathy.

## Futile treatments

**The prevailing creed or buzzword in patients with diabetic feet is 'salvage'.** Vast energies and resources are invested in the 'salvage the limb campaign' — an obsession that often leads to futile care. I see examples of such cases all around — **below is a typical one**.

> An 84-year-old, obese, diabetic man with the usual comorbidities. He can hardly walk around the house with a walker. He develops a DFU with osteomyelitis of the great toe, which is then amputated. The stump does not heal. Toe pressures are 'borderline'. Vascular surgery orders a CT angio, which demonstrates multisegmental arterial disease, and the patient undergoes multiple stent insertions. Foot perfusion improves, but the 2nd and 3rd toes also develop ulcers. Podiatry performs forefoot (transmetatarsal) amputation, following which the leg and foot become dusky. Back to vascular surgery — now thrombolysis of the occluded stents is needed. The foot stump becomes necrotic. The patient becomes septic and is transferred to the university hospital, where he undergoes a below-knee amputation. Five days later, he is discharged to a nursing home. The below-knee stump falls apart and doesn't heal despite prolonged wound care by various 'wound care experts'. The patient is admitted to the hospital for above-knee amputation, following which he develops acute-on-chronic renal failure requiring dialysis. Meanwhile, he develops a sacral decubitus ulcer and a large pressure ulcer on the heel of the remaining foot. A 'wound care expert' is summoned...

**Sounds like a 'nightmare', right? But such 'nightmares' are so common. Try to imagine such a 9-month saga, which commonly ends in death.** The multiple hospitalizations, the days spent driving to the various clinics, the days of work lost to the family members, and the huge expenses. **And there is no one around to take leadership and decide when enough is enough, to suggest that an 'early amputation' at the proper, well-perfused level, achieving a well-healed stump, is preferable to prolonged sagas of suffering and futility.**

**Well, perhaps you, the wound care specialist, who spends weeks with the patient and his family trying to heal his non-healing wound, are better positioned to discuss potential futility!**

**"You should consider the feet and toes of a diabetic patient as a 'time bomb'. What you see on the 'outside' is like the tip of the iceberg — beneath the innocuous-looking plantar callus, the bone may be chewed up with infection."**

# Chapter 15

## Ischemic ulcers

*Whatever is the etiology of the wound, always suspect and evaluate for overt or latent underlying ischemia.*

Another term for **ischemic ulcers** is **arterial ulcers**, to distinguish them from **venous ulcers**, which are caused by a different mechanism of ischemia (➲ Chapters 2 and 13). **In most cases, your job here is to correctly diagnose the ischemic nature of the ulcer and refer to your surgical friends for the restoration of arterial circulation (hopefully) or amputation**. In selected cases, you will only palliate or 'maintain' the ulcer.

The majority of cases are caused by atherosclerosis-related **peripheral vascular disease** (PVD). **Arterial embolism** (discussed separately below) is a much rarer etiology, whereas wounds caused by **vasculitis** are so infrequent that it is unlikely you will be encountering any.

**Don't forget that many ischemic ulcers are 'mixed'** — diabetic ulcers can be 'ischemic' as well, pressure ulcers can develop in ischemic feet, and arterial ischemia can affect patients with underlying chronic venous stasis. Of course, morbidly obese patients can suffer from all these components together.

### Clinical features

**The patient is typically an older male with well-known risk factors** (e.g. smoking, diabetes) and associated comorbidities (e.g. ischemic heart disease, carotid artery disease). Some — those who still walk around — would give you a history of **intermittent claudication** (pain in the calf during walking). **But**

**when significant tissue ischemia develops, the pain becomes steady ('rest pain'), which tends to increase when the leg is elevated** (remember? — the opposite situation to venous ulcers).

**Ninety-nine percent of ischemic ulcers affect the lower limb**. Naturally, distal tissues, supplied by 'end arteries' are most susceptible. **Ulcers developing on the tip of the toes (unlike the diabetic ulcers situated on the base, at pressure points) are characteristic. Other areas commonly affected are on the top, and lateral aspect of the feet.**

## Examination

**The following are typical findings**:

- **Ulcers are well-demarcated — 'punched-out'**. They are painful as opposed to diabetic ulcers. They are pale or gangrenous. Patients can present with acute on chronic ischemia (■ Figure 15.1), or chronic ischemia (■ Figure 15.2).

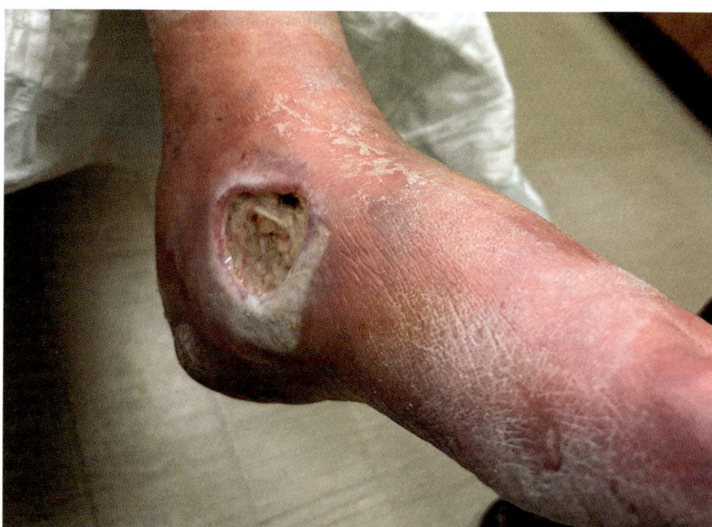

Figure 15.1. An ischemic ulcer in a patient presenting with critical limb ischemia — punched out, pale; some exudate; the whole limb is cyanotic.

- **The surrounding skin reflects chronic ischemia**: pale or cyanotic, with hair loss.

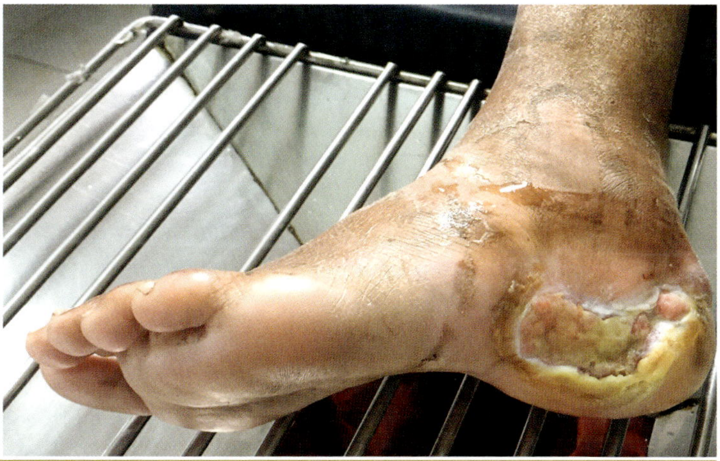

Figure 15.2. An ischemic ulcer in a patient with chronic limb ischemia — punched out, pale, dry; the limb is pale.

- **Gangrene can extend to the periwound**. It can be 'dry' or 'wet' (■ Figure 15.3).

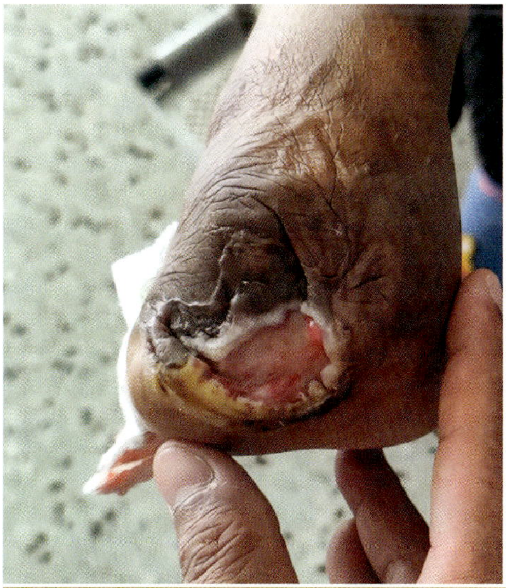

Figure 15.3. An ischemic ulcer developing in a forefoot amputation stump. Note the gangrenous periwound.

- **Peripheral pulses. Palpable foot pulses exclude the ischemic etiology of the ulcer**. It is, however, not always true in diabetic patients or in some cases of emboli occluding the arteries of the toes (see below). **Now don't be lazy — roll down the patient's heavy blue jeans and assess the femoral and popliteal pulses**, which are easier to palpate than the foot pulses in swollen legs. The absence of those pulses is diagnostic for significant PVD.

**Demonstrate that you are a solid clinician and perform the following simple tests**:

- **Elevation pallor**: elevate the leg to 60° and watch the color of the soles of the feet. No change should occur in normally perfused feet. Pallor appearing within 30 seconds indicates significant arterial disease. Mild and moderate ischemia will appear within 40 to 60 seconds.
- **Dependency rubor**: now let the foot hang down and wait a minute or so. Significant arterial disease will manifest when the foot turns dusky red. It is caused by compensatory vasodilation of the skin microvasculature. The rubor will subside when you elevate the foot.
- **Capillary refill**: press firmly on the tip of the great toe until the skin blanches; now release the pressure and observe the color of the toe. It should normalize within 2-3 seconds. Prolonged recovery suggests some degree of ischemia.

## Diagnosis

I have mentioned already, the various investigations used to assess leg perfusion in ➲ Chapter 4. **Below are some more details**.

### ABIs

**As you know already, the measurement of the ABI is integral in the assessment of all sorts of leg wounds.** ■ Table 15.1 shows the spectrum of ABIs and their clinical significance:

- **In the context of wound care, an ABI of 0.5-0.9 suggests 'relative ischemia'** — not the direct cause of the ulcer or wound — but a factor which could be preventing wound healing. It is not what we are discussing in this chapter.
- **An ABI of <0.5 signifies CRITICAL LIMB ISCHEMIA, causing 'rest pain' and/or tissue loss (ulceration and/or gangrene). It is the situation typified by ischemic ulcers.**

**Table 15.1. Ankle-Brachial Index (ABI).**

| ABI | Significance |
|---|---|
| >1.3 | Non-compressible (calcified vessels) typical in diabetic patients<br>Look at toe pressures (➡ Chapter 14) |
| 0.9-1.3 | Normal |
| 0.5-0.9 | Mild to moderate PVD; intermittent claudication can be present |
| <0.5 | Critical limb ischemia leading to rest pain, ulceration and/or gangrene |

### Non-invasive imaging

In the setting of **critical limb ischemia**, when the patient must be referred urgently to vascular surgery, you'd better let the 'experts' order the tests of their choice, i.e. duplex ultrasound, CT angiography (CTA), MR angiography (MRA) to better delineate the vascular pathology and plan options for revascularization.

In 'less urgent' cases, for example, a patient with a diabetic foot, when I am not sure how 'ischemic' their diabetic ulcer is, I may order a CTA.

## Treatment

**There is not much to discuss here about wound care, as patients with critical limb ischemia belong to the vascular surgeon. Let the surgeon decide about revascularization procedures or amputation.**

**There is no point in debriding an ischemic wound because it is not going to heal.** So, just apply to the wound some topical antiseptic such as povidone iodine (Betadine®), or silver sulfadiazine (SSD™) cream, and a dressing, start antibiotics (if necessary), and talk to the vascular surgeon.

**How urgent is the situation?**

- **Emergency**: ulcers associated with major foot and/or leg gangrene require emergency treatment; **more so when the gangrene is 'wet' — signifying life-threatening invasive infection**.
- **Urgent**: on the other hand, ischemic ulcers without surrounding gangrene or with localized dry gangrene do not need to be 'shipped out' immediately. A delay of a day or two would be reasonable.

**Some of these patients will be returned to your wound care clinic for one of the following reasons**:

- The surgeon decides that revascularization is unfeasible.
- The patient declines amputation.
- After successful revascularization, to manage the original, now better-perfused wound.
- After amputation, to manage the amputation wounds, which often break down.

**Other patients may return after revascularization, with dry gangrene involving the toes. (Those with wet gangrene would have been amputated.) In general, there is no need to debride the dry gangrene — let it 'demarcate' and fall off spontaneously; let the toe 'auto-amputate'**. However, keep monitoring the wound as occasionally the 'dry' gangrene may turn 'wet' and require debridement/amputation of the involved part.

## Compression in ischemic limbs?

I mentioned it already in ➲ Chapter 8. When the ABI is >0.8, compression is safe. In patients with an ABI of 0.5-0.8, use 'lighter' compression (20-30mmHg). **In patients with critical limb ischemia, the rule is 'no compression until revascularization'. However, any rule has exceptions**: what to do with, say, in a patient with an ischemic ulcer and an ABI of 0.5, with a swollen leg, who cannot be revascularized or awaits an appointment with the vascular surgeon? I would compress him very lightly ('as tolerated') with a Tubigrip®. ***Remember* — any compression is better than no compression**.

## Embolic skin ulcers

Skin ulcers due to ischemic injury caused by emboli is rare. But you have to be aware of them as they herald a life-threatening situation needing urgent medical attention.

## Pathophysiology

**Ulceration develops when embolic particles occlude the small arterioles supplying the skin, causing localized necrosis and ulcers.**

We are not talking here about **macro embolism** — large pieces of clot (the most common source being the heart in patients with atrial fibrillation) lodged in **large and medium-sized arteries**, resulting in acute critical limb ischemia, which indicates an emergency vascular intervention.

**Instead, what we are talking about are microemboli — tiny pieces of cholesterol crystals detached from ulcerated atherosclerotic plaques in proximal major vessels such as the aorta (e.g. aortic arch and abdominal aortic aneurysms) — also called atheroemboli.** Atheroembolism can be spontaneous in patients with advanced atherosclerosis. It can also occur following invasive vascular procedures, which injure or disturb the plaques. **Paradoxically, anticoagulation can also precipitate atheroemboli by inducing intra-plaque hemorrhage or impairing the healing of an ulcerated plaque.**

## Clinical features

The presentation may be acute or insidious. More than one toe (in both feet) can be affected. The toe turns blue or purple; gradually, over a few days, the affected skin undergoes necrosis and/or ulceration. **This is why the condition is termed 'blue toe syndrome'.** The pain is usually out of proportion to the clinical findings. **The foot itself is often well perfused, with palpable pulses — don't let this finding confuse you!**

**Diagnosis requires a high level of suspicion**: suggestive clinical features developing in patients with a history of atherosclerosis, aortic aneurysm, anticoagulants, or a recent vascular procedure are suggestive.

## Treatment

Initially, the management of the ischemic toes is secondary. **What is more important is to establish the source of the microemboli and prevent further tissue injury.** Additional diagnostic and therapeutic decisions do not fall within the scope of the wound care clinic.

**"Here are the 5 Ps of limb ischemia: Pain, Pallor, Pulselessness, Paresthesia, Paralysis. But the limb can be ischemic even if none of these signs are present."**

# Chapter 16

## Pressure ulcers

*If he has a bedsore, it's generally not the fault of the disease, but of the nursing.*

**Florence Nightingale (1820-1910)**

**Pressure ulcers, or whatever you choose to call them (pressure wounds, bed sores, pressure injuries), are prevalent**: each year, more than 3 million cases are treated in the USA. You will meet them in acute care hospitals, nursing homes, wound care clinics, and at home.

### Pathophysiology

**Sustained pressure high enough to occlude capillary blood flow (~30mmHg) can initiate ischemic tissue injury within 1-2 hours. Immobility is the key etiologic factor** — if the person moves, if they can change position (or someone helps them) in the bed or wheelchair every hour or so, then a pressure ulcer won't develop. Here are a few points:

- **Common sites of pressure ulcers are depicted in ■ Figure 16.1.** They represent 'bony' areas where the skin is 'squeezed' between the external pressure and the underlying bones. Which sites are involved depends on the patient's position (e.g. **sacrum**, **coccyx**, and **heels** in supine, bedridden patients; **greater trochanters** when lying on one side; **ischial tuberosities** in sitting patients). **Morbidly obese patients** are susceptible because of the increased pressure generated by their weight. However, **cachectic patients** are also vulnerable, as they have lost the subcutaneous padding of their skin.

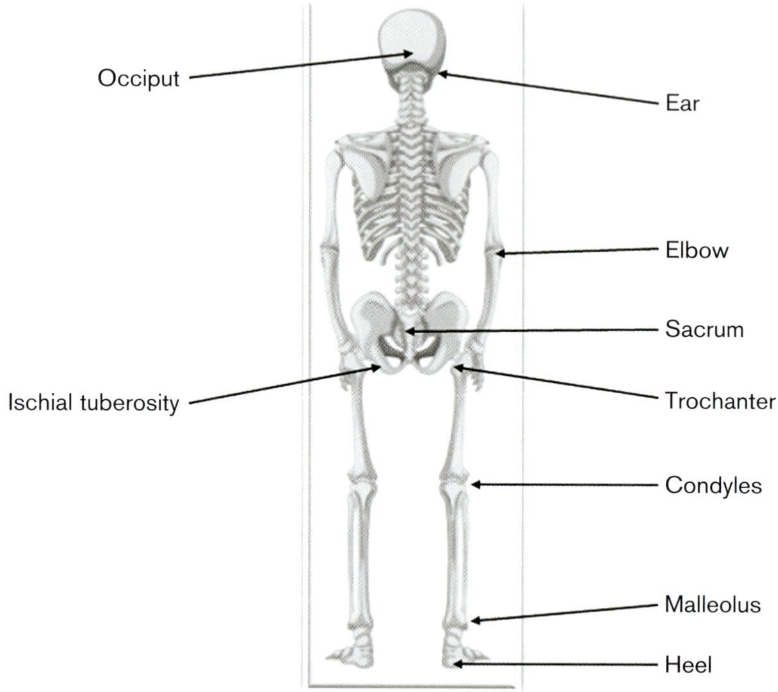


**Figure 16.1. Common sites of pressure ulcers.**

- **Medical devices can cause pressure injury**: a cast applied too tightly to the leg, an improperly secured nasogastric tube causing an ulcer at the tip of the nose, or a wrongly managed urinary catheter ulcerating the tip of the penis.

**It's not only immobility**. Other factors producing or contributing to skin injury are:

- **Shear forces**: when the skin is stretched away from the underlying tissue. It occurs when the patient's body slides down in their bed or wheelchair.
- **Friction**: repeated friction of the skin against another surface. Think about the heel of a paraplegic patient constantly banging against the wheelchair. Or the hammertoe of an old lady rubbing against her shoe. **In fact, pressure or friction injury plays a significant role in diabetic foot ulcers!**
- **Excessive moisture**: excessively moist skin is especially susceptible to pressure injury. Think about the incontinent older man lying unattended for hours in a pool of feces and urine. Or the fat guy sitting in a wheelchair with a constantly sweating buttock.

## Assessment

I mentioned already that I don't like the various staging or grading systems of wounds. Too many systems are described and this is confusing. **One exception is the staging system of pressure ulcers, which, believe it or not, I use constantly.** ■ Table 16.1 describes and explains the various stages.

**Table 16.1. Stages of pressure ulcers.**

| Stage | Description | Comments |
|---|---|---|
| **I** | **Non-blanchable erythema**. The involved skin area doesn't turn pale when you press/release on it with the finger. | Consider it as a 'pre-ulcer'. If the pressure is not relieved rapidly, injury can progress to stage II within a day. |
| **II** | **Partial-thickness skin loss. The dermis is exposed but not subcutaneous fat**. It can start as a blister. | |
| **III** | **Full-thickness skin loss. The subcutaneous fat is exposed but *not* the muscle, tendon or bone.** | |
| **IV** | **Full-thickness skin loss with exposed muscle, tendon or bone.** | It can be associated with osteomyelitis of the exposed bone. |
| **Unstageable** | **The surface of the wound is obscured by slough or eschar**. You can assess the stage only after thorough debridement. | ➲ Figure 16.2. |
| **Deep tissue injury** | **Persistent dark red, maroon or purple discoloration, overlying a 'lumpy', firm or boggy area**. It indicates significant pressure injury to the soft tissues residing between the skin and bone. | Even after immediate offloading of the involved area, the overlying skin may break down and progress to stages II, III, or IV. |

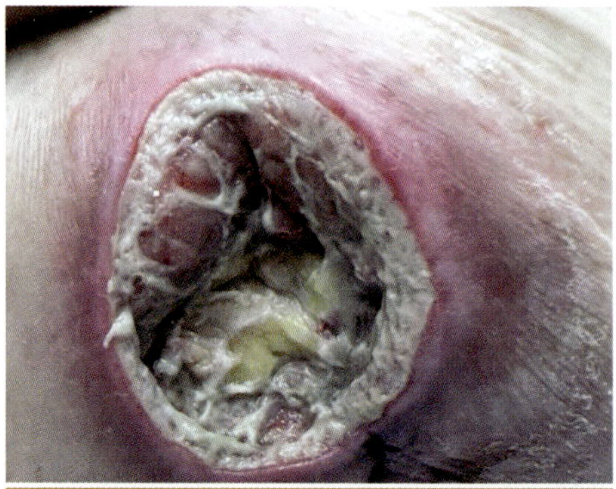

Figure 16.2. Unstageable sacral ulcer. What's hiding behind the slough?

**As you can see, assessment of pressure ulcers is primarily clinical.** In non-healing stage IV ulcers, an MRI may be necessary to diagnose osteomyelitis, which can be confirmed with a bone biopsy.

## Treatment

The two components in the treatment of pressure ulcers are:

- **Offloading the injured skin area. It applies to all ulcer stages.**
- **Wound management** (according to the principles described in ➲ Part II).

**Let's now look at each stage separately:**

- **Stage I: this is a warning sign.** If detected and properly managed, progression to ulceration can be prevented. **Offloading is the key: the rule of thumb is to stay off the area until it returns to normal.** Bedridden patients should be repositioned at least every 2 hours; in a wheelchair, they should be helped to shift position every 15 minutes. Air-, fluid-, or gel-filled mattresses are recommended to relieve and distribute pressure. Doughnut-style cushions are *not* recommended as they can produce pressure injury to the periwound. **The injured area** should be gently washed with soap and water and dried. It should be covered with **moisture barrier creams** (e.g. zinc, petroleum), or a **protective dressing** (e.g. a hydrocolloid like DuoDERM®), which also provides cushioning.

- **Stage II: these are shallow, full-thickness ulcers and thus they rarely require debridement**. Which dressings should you use? I like to place a few drops of honey onto the wound, covered with a bordered foam dressing (e.g. Mepilex®). But anything will work, provided the wound is kept clean and moist, the periwound is well maintained, and, above all, offloading is perfect.
- **Stage III: in these full-thickness ulcers, the exposed subcutaneous fat is often necrotic and in need of debridement. In most cases, you can proceed with 'selective-conservative' debridement** at the bedside without anesthesia (➲ Chapter 5). Excise the non-viable tissue piece-meal until healthy bleeding tissue is encountered. Repeat it as many times as needed. Follow with the 'standard wound care' (➲ Chapters 5, 6, 7 and 8).
- **Stage IV: the base of these deep ulcers is usually composed of necrotic tissue, slough, and pus. Exposed bone is often palpable. The skin edges are commonly undermined and non-viable. Tunneling is common** (■ Figure 16.3). **Thus, proper surgical debridement is indicated to control sepsis and produce a healable wound, either spontaneously or in preparation for subsequent operative reconstruction**. The procedure may include debridement of the underlying bone. It is a major surgical procedure performed in the operating room. Subsequently, re-debridement, which is often required, can be 'selective' at the bedside.

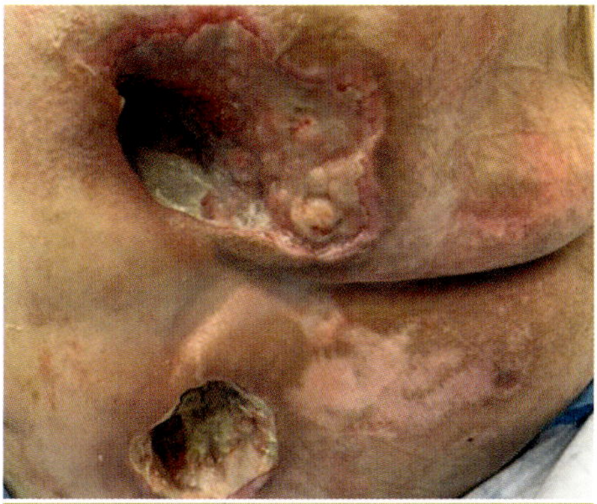

**Figure 16.3. Stage IV, tunneling sacral ulcer managed successfully with negative pressure wound therapy (NPWT).**

**Wound care is demanding, requiring ingenuity**, paying attention to keeping the cavities and tunnels well drained. **Negative pressure wound**

**therapy (NPWT) is beneficial for treating deep, complex wounds** (➲ Chapter 9). The 'VAC' dressing has to be conformed to the specific wound location (e.g. sacrum, heel). You don't want the patient to lie on the pressure-sensing pad and tubing, which can cause additional pressure injuries. **The solution is to create a 'bridge' — a long strip of foam interposed between the foam in the wound and the remote, desired location for the pressure sensing pad and the tubing**. You can fashion the 'bridge' by yourself or use one of the commercial pre-made bridges available (e.g. 3M GranuFoam Bridge™).

**For an unstageable pressure injury**, selective and conservative bedside debridement of all non-viable tissue will expose the base of the wound to become stageable. Remember, however, not to debride the dry eschar on the heel as shown in ■ Figure 16.4 (➲ Chapter 5) or on an ischemic limb (➲ Chapter 15).

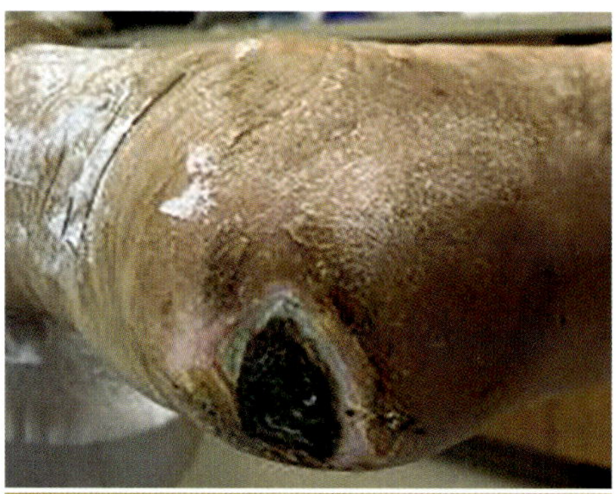

**Figure 16.4. Unstageable heel ulcer. Leave the dry eschar alone!**

**For a deep tissue injury**, the management is limited to offloading and protecting the injured area with suitable dressings. There is nothing to cut out. Just let the extent of the injury declare itself within a few days.

## Prevention

**"If he has a bedsore, it's generally not the fault of the disease, but of the nursing.**" This adage is attributed to **Florence Nightingale** (1820-1910), the British founder of modern nursing. She described proper preventive measures, including the advice to "inspect every nook and cranny" of the skin. It appears, however, that nothing has changed since then — preventive measures are detailed in the curriculum of nursing schools, in protocols of hospitals and nursing homes, and in numerous guidelines of various societies. **Still, pressure injuries are as common as before**. As you know, prevention is secondary in our flailing medical industry, where the emphasis is on 'treating' rather than preventing — **hospitals and providers are not compensated for preventing a bed sore; they are, however, for the debridement of the sores**…

I believe that most of you, as 'wound care providers', with your background in nursing or medicine, are well familiar with the preventive measures. These include:

- **Offloading**: pressure redistribution, frequent repositioning (in bed or in a wheelchair), using specialized mattresses or cushions.
- **Protecting susceptible pressure points**.
- **Skin care**: clean, proper moisture control.
- **Mobility enhancement**.
- **Adequate nutrition and hydration**.

**In brief, your job is not only to treat the pressure wound but also to determine why it developed and to educate the patient and those who care for them on how to prevent similar injuries**. Talk to the nursing home staff, inspect the patient's shoes, and be sure that they are not constantly bumping their heels against the wheelchair. You know the spiel!

**"Pressure wounds: easy to prevent, so hard to heal."**

# Chapter 17

## Post-surgical wounds

*In a perfect world all post-surgical wounds are the operating surgeon's responsibility. But the world is not perfect...*

In your wound care clinic, you will encounter numerous patients with postoperative wounds. In ➲ Chapter 2, I have explained why you are seeing these patients rather than the surgeons who created the wounds. **The spectrum of such wounds is as broad as the spectrum of operations performed by the various surgical specialties**. You may see, for example:

- A 'simple' abdominal wound infection developing a week after the patient was discharged from 'St. Elsewhere'.
- A chronically festering wound with an underlying infected mesh following a hernia repair a year ago.
- A draining thigh sinus leading to the infected hardware following hip replacement.
- A large wound following extensive debridement of necrotizing fasciitis (■ Figure 17.1).

**The range of possible scenarios is endless.**

**My advice: share responsibility**. Contact the surgeon who performed the original operation. Ask him or her what they want to do. Do they want to take the patient back? If not, or if the case involved 'itinerant surgery' — the bariatric procedure operation was performed in Mexico, or in some 'ivory tower' hundreds of miles away — speak to your local surgeons. **Let them decide what images the patient needs and how to continue their care.**

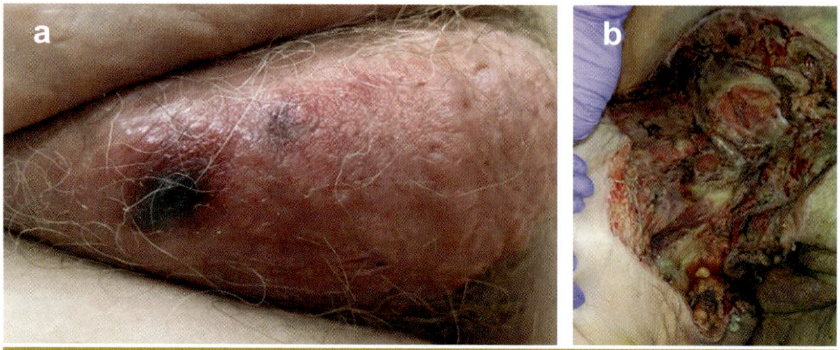

Figure 17.1. a) A diabetic patient presenting with necrotizing fasciitis of the mons pubis spreading to the lower abdomen and groin. b) After radical debridement the wound was treated with a 'wound VAC'.

**One more point: if, after removing the dressings, you see exposed hardware, vessels, or grafts, consider it an emergency**. Reapply a fresh dressing and ship the patient out!

Of course, you will be dealing with many postoperative patients referred to you by the local surgeons to take over long-term wound care. A typical example is a non-healing foot or leg amputation performed for diabetic feet or peripheral arterial disease (■ Figure 17.2).

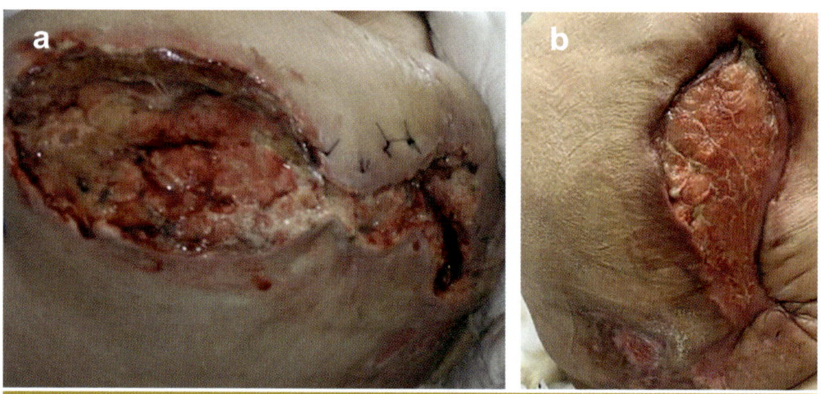

Figure 17.2. a) A dehisced, infected above-knee amputation stump. b) After debridement and prolonged treatment with a 'wound VAC'.

**"Share responsibility with your local surgeon. Otherwise — if something goes wrong — the original surgeon will blame you for his complication!"**

# Chapter 18

## Post-traumatic wounds and hematomas

*Doubt as to the condition of the wound should incline one to pessimism rather than to mistaken optimism.*

**William Heneage Ogilvie, 1887-1971**

Of course, your wound care clinic is not a trauma center or an emergency room. Therefore, you are not going to encounter wounds in the acute stage. The wounds that you will see are:

- Wounds which were already treated, but failed to heal, as expected after say a week or two, or more.
- Wounds that were untreated for some reason — commonly neglected by the patient.

Most of these patients would have already received a course or two of antibiotics, indicated or not, from their primary care providers.

The mechanism of injury to the soft tissues could be diverse — laceration, avulsion, crush, degloving, puncture — but it doesn't matter much at the stage when the patient presents to you. In the literature, you will find a whole host of **grading systems** for trauma wounds that incorporate factors such as type, size, depth, and extent of tissue loss. But practically, I find such systems only of academic interest — for us, a wound is a wound, and you describe and deal with what you see (➲ Chapter 4).

## Why do these wounds fail to heal?

By now, you surely know the spiel (➲ Chapter 3, ■ Table 3.2): patient- and wound-related factors are the same. But in my experience, **iatrogenic factors play a significant role in the context of post-traumatic wounds**, where many wounds are treated inappropriately in emergency rooms or doctors' offices by non-surgeons. Thus, for example:

- **Wounds that should be left open are sutured**: think about the neglected dog bite wound on the arm, which was sutured in the ER with resulting gross wound infection. Or the degloving injury on the leg, where the ER doc attempted to suture the non-viable thin skin flap, which becomes necrotic after a few days. **Such wounds should have been left open for spontaneous healing**.
- **Wounds which were repaired with a faulty technique**: inadequate debridement of non-viable tissue; inadequate removal of 'foreign matter' (e.g. tiny pieces of glass, dirt); failure to obliterate dead space (i.e. closing the skin but neglecting the gaping subcutaneous fat and/or muscle); failure to leave a drain, if needed; closure under excessive tension.
- **Skin sutures or staplers removed prematurely**. A plastic surgeon does a beautiful wound reconstruction after excision of a skin cancer. The patient is sent home with the instructions, "remove the sutures after 7 days". Then, when a nurse removes the sutures in an office, the wound opens up.

## Treatment

The management of these wounds follows the basics described in ➲ Part II. Here are a few points:

- The first thing to do is to remove all residual sutures and staplers that may still be hanging out or embedded in the wound.
- Debride all non-viable tissue, including old scabs, loose non-viable skin edges or flaps, and drain old blood or pus (■ Figures 18.1 and 18.2).
- Wound care and management of infection (if suspected) — as described earlier in the book.
- If the wound appears too 'deep' or too 'complex' for your abilities, then ask for the help of a surgeon.

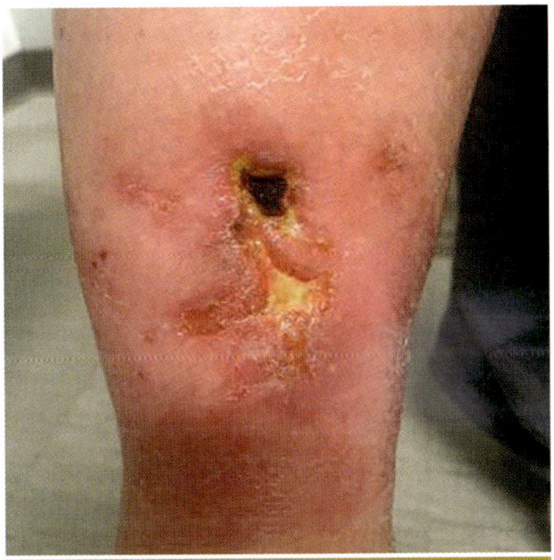

Figure 18.1. A 3-week-old, superficially penetrating wound of the thigh in a swollen leg. There was pus under the eschar, causing the surrounding cellulitis.

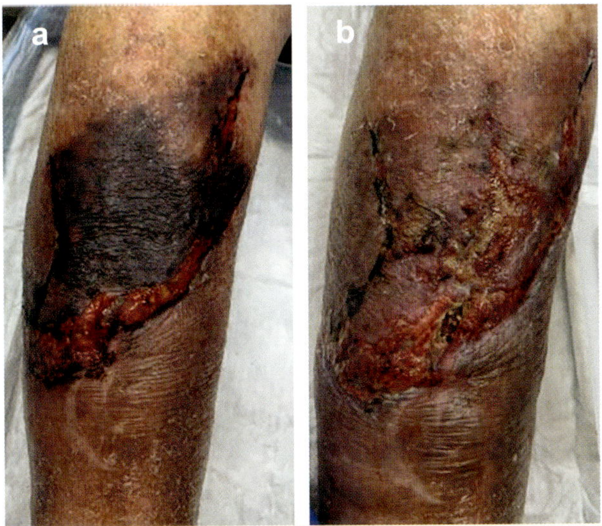

Figure 18.2. A 2-week-old degloving wound of the shin. a) At presentation — note the necrotic skin flap which had been sutured in the ER (sutures now removed). b) Two weeks after debridement and treatment with honey.

## Hematomas

**Soft tissue hematomas developing after blunt trauma are a common cause of complex open wounds. I have already raised this issue in ➲ Chapter 2, but here are a few more words.**

Yes, the 'traditional' approach to post-traumatic hematomas of the extremities is conservative, unless they are expanding rapidly and/or there are features of compartment syndrome (e.g. neurovascular compromise of the extremity). The conventional teaching is that such hematomas will resolve spontaneously over weeks to months (depending on their size). Thus, the common trend in the 'community' is to temporize.

**So, the older guy on warfarin, who develops a knee hematoma after falling, is seen in the ER**. The X-ray reports "only soft tissue swelling". He is discharged; "it will resolve, just elevate your leg", he is being told. Occasionally, someone is smart enough to discontinue the warfarin; often not. At home, **the local swelling increases** due to ongoing bleeding, inflammation, or the 'expanding process' where blood breakdown products create high osmotic pressure, drawing fluid into the space. After a week, the patient consults his primary care provider, who describes a "large bluish swelling" and reassures the patient that "it will resolve — be patient".

**A few days later, the local pain increases**, and the patient returns to the ER. An ultrasound is ordered, describing "a complex subcutaneous fluid collection, most likely a hematoma". Yet again, the patient is reassured — *don't we know that the management of hematomas is conservative?* **A week later, the primary care doc observes darkening of the skin overlying the swelling and refers the patient to a surgeon. Now the surgeon debrides the necrotic skin and evacuates the hematoma, producing a large cavity and wound which needs many weeks of management** (■ Figure 18.3).

**The message is clear: whereas the initial approach to soft tissue hematomas is 'conservative', these patients should undergo careful, frequent follow-up**. When the skin stretched over the bulging mass becomes tender, discolored (or insensate), it means that it's compromised — the hematoma should be urgently drained before the skin dies!

**At this stage, the procedure is simple**: place a small incision at the center of the bulge, squeeze the clots out, irrigate the cavity, and apply a tight compression dressing to prevent the reaccumulation of fluid in the

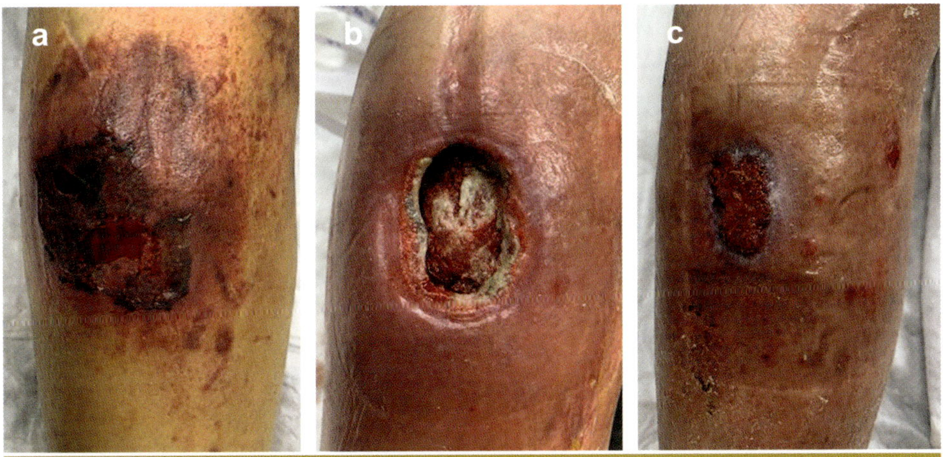

**Figure 18.3. Post-traumatic hematoma overlying the knee. a) Presentation. b) The wound after evacuation of the hematoma and debridement (note the significant undermining of the skin edges). c) After 5 weeks of treatment with a 'wound VAC'.**

cavity. Two days later, expose the wound, squeeze out any remaining clots/fluid, and compress again. **You have saved the patient from a prolonged morbidity!**

## Burns

**From time to time, patients with burns will show up at your clinic a few days after the accident**. The vast majority of burns are thermal (e.g. hot fluids, direct heat source); chemical or electrical burns are rare. The types of burns treated in your outpatient settings range from very superficial injuries to deeper burns that can still heal without immediate surgical intervention. **These are mostly 'minor' or 'moderate' burns, as the 'major' burns will have been referred to dedicated 'burn centers'**.

**The management of 'minor' burns is straightforward — you can deal with them. However, you must assess and decide whether you can/should manage the 'moderate' burns rather than refer them to a specialist (e.g. a burn center or hand surgeon)**.

**But first, let's remind ourselves of some basic definitions — how do we 'classify' burns? How do we decide what's 'minor' vs. 'moderate' vs. 'major'?** You will hear or read about many terms used to describe burns: 'first degree', 'second degree', and so forth; 'superficial' vs. 'deep'; 'partial thickness' vs. 'full thickness'. Let us tie all those terms into a workable narrative.

## Staging of burns

**The staging of burns is predominantly based on their depth:**

- **First-degree (superficial) burns**: these involve the epidermis only. The skin is erythematous, dry and painful. There are no blisters. It heals within a few days. Severe sun burn is an example. **You won't be seeing these cases in your clinic**.
- **Second-degree burns**: these involve the dermis to various depths:
  - **superficial second-degree (partial-thickness)**: these involve the upper layer of the dermis. The area is very painful (sensate!), pink, moist, it blanches briskly and there are blisters. **With optimal care it will heal within 2 weeks with no or only minimal scarring or some pigmentation**;
  - **deep second-degree (partial-thickness)**: these extend into the deeper (reticular) dermis. The area appears mottled or 'waxy' with reduced blanching. It's less painful and sensation is present but altered. Eschar can develop within a few days. Healing by epithelization takes 3 weeks or longer. **Scar formation is common — especially when healing is prolonged**. **Second-degree burns are the ones you will mainly see in the clinic**.
- **Third-degree burns (full-thickness)**: the whole epidermis and dermis are destroyed. The involved area is white, brown or charred, non-blanching and insensate. **Eschar forms rapidly**. Because the burn destroys all skin adnexa (e.g. hair follicles, sweat glands, sebaceous glands) — the source of epithelial cells which regenerate the skin in partial thickness-thickness burns — **spontaneous healing is by epithelial migration from the wound edges and contraction, resulting in obligatory scarring**. **Most such burns do not belong to the wound care clinic, unless very small, in 'non-critical' cosmetic sites**.
- **Fourth-degree burns (full-thickness)**: these extend into the subcutaneous fat and beyond, into muscle or bone. The area is charred, black, obviously insensate. **These are 'surgical cases' — not for your wound care clinic**.

**Note that areas of burn are often of 'mixed-degree'**; for example, a second-degree burn with a small area at its center exhibiting features of a third-degree burn. A 'mix' of first-degree, superficial second-degree, and deep second-degree burns is common.

**Remember also that the location of the burns matters**: a deep second-degree burn resulting in a scar on the dorsum of the hand is of little significance, but a scar overlying the finger joints could result in contractures and loss of function; and a scar on the face in a younger lady would be a cosmetic disaster.

## Total body surface area (TBSA) of burns

**The TBSA** (**excluding first-degree burns!**) **has a crucial impact on the outcome and treatment**. For example, involvement of >20% of the skin surface represents a 'major' burn and would be shipped to the burn center. **So, how do we estimate TBSA?**

I don't bother much with TBSA in the wound clinic. The patient's TBSA has already been estimated in the emergency room (usually using the 'rule of nines'), so it doesn't matter much to me whether it's 1% or 3%. **If I do, I use the 'palm method': the skin area corresponding to the patient's palm (including the fingers) represents ~1% of TBSA**. Such a method is practical for the minor, irregular, scattered burns we often see in the clinic. Eyeballing the burns, one can estimate that the total surface involved is, say, '3 palms', which translates to 3%.

## 'Minor' vs. 'moderate' vs. 'major' burns

Now, you can combine all the information above ('degree' of burn, location and TBSA) and decide whether the burn is 'minor', 'moderate' or 'major':

- **Minor burns**: these include all first-degree burns and small (<10% TBSA) second-degree burns that don't involve **'problem' areas** such as the face, feet, genitalia, perineum, and major joints. **They can be managed in your wound care clinic**.
- **Moderate burns**: these are second-degree burns of between 10-20% TBSA, and some smaller second-degree burns affecting 'problem' areas. **They can be managed in your wound care clinic, depending on your resources. Some may need the help of a 'specialist'**.

- **Major burns**: these include second-degree burns of >20% TBSA or any significant third-degree burns (>1-2%). Included are also deep second-degree burns involving 'problem' areas as well as all electrical, chemical burns, circumferential limb burns (risk of compartment syndrome), circumferential chest burns and inhalation injury (risk of respiratory distress). **You won't be dealing with them.**

## Treatment of burns

As with wound care in general, people use different treatment options based on questionable levels of evidence. **Here are my recommendations.**

- **First-degree burns**: clean with cool running water and mild soap. Apply an emollient lotion, such as petroleum jelly (e.g. Vaseline®), or another neutral (unscented, no alcohol) moisturizing agent. Leave open or cover with any simple dressing. Repeat as above daily. **Please — there is no need for any topical antimicrobial agent!**
- **Second-degree burns**: these wounds are painful and require oral analgesia. **Systemic antibiotics** should be given only if clear features of bacterial superinfection develop during the treatment (rare!). **Local care depends on the depth of the burn, with its characteristic findings**:
  - **debridement: blisters (typical of the 'superficial' form) should be punctured and completely unroofed**, to allow contact of the dressing with the healing dermis. **Eschar** — the dry, firm, dark layer of non-viable tissue adherent to the wound bed, which tends to develop within a few days on the 'deep' second-degree burn, should be removed as well. True, you could wait for it to fall off on its own, but it would take weeks and increase the risk of infection developing under it and of scarring. Hence, I remove it ASAP —often piecemeal over a week or so. After a few days, it becomes loose and easily peels off with sterile forceps. The process is relatively painless as the 'deep' second-degree burns have reduced sensation;
  - **dressings**: the 'chaos' described in previous chapters concerning the selection of dressings pertains to burn care as well. **Historically, silver sulfadiazine (SSD™) cream**, with its broad antimicrobial activity to prevent infection, was the most recommended agent for the treatment of burns. **Its low cost, widespread availability, and ease of use still make it the most widely used agent for burns worldwide.** After cleansing the area, apply a thin layer of SSD™, cover with a non-adherent, paraffin-impregnated dressing (e.g. Jelonet®), and use a secondary

dressing (gauze would do). However, the emerging 'fashion' is to move away from this simple method towards more 'fancy' options, based on claims that SSD™ delays healing. **Thus, the current trend is to use one of the modern silver-impregnated occlusive dressings** (see ➲ Chapter 7), **which do not need frequent changes**. Some people like to apply a topical antibiotic (e.g. mupirocin) on burns, but this is unnecessary unless a culture-proven staphylococcal infection is documented. **And let us not forget that honey** (➲ Chapter 6) **has been proven to be an excellent option for the treatment of second-degree burns: apply a generous layer of honey and cover with your secondary dressing of choice**.

**A few more points**:

- **'Deep' second-degree burns take longer to heal. The longer the healing time, the higher the risk of scarring and contractures**. Thus, if no healing occurs by the end of 3 weeks, consider referring to a surgeon for excision and skin grafting, especially if the burns are extensive or involve the hands, joints, or face.
- **The same applies to the minor, isolated third-degree burns** that you may elect to treat. The one in a non-functional area, you may leave to scar down or refer out.

**Burns are just wounds. So apply the usual concepts of wound care: remove what's non-viable, prevent/treat infection, and provide 'moist' wound treatment**.

**"If you treat a complicated wound you get wound complications."**

# Chapter 19

## Morbid obesity-related wounds

*The fatter he is, the more complex are his wounds, and the more demanding is the wound care required.*

**I have already mentioned (➲ Chapter 2) that the obese and morbidly obese are frequent fliers in our wound care clinics**, with wounds resulting from a complex interplay of physiological, mechanical, and vascular factors.

**The most common condition that brings the morbidly obese patient to my wound care clinic is 'swollen, ulcerated, weeping legs'**. These patients suffer from chronic stasis dermatitis (➲ Chapters 2 and 8); they do not, or cannot, use adequate compression (➲ Chapter 8). Minor skin injuries do not heal. Cellulitis sets in, and the leg balloons; ulcers pop up, and leak profusely, soaking their dressing. **They are miserable!**

You already know how to help these patients: **wound care** — moisture control, appropriate dressings, and antibiotics (when indicated); **optimal compression** — e.g. Unna boots, Profore®. **And when the acute situation resolves**, the legs dry out and return to baseline — ensure they can wear long-term compression garments to prevent recurrence (e.g. one of the easy-to-use Velcro compression wraps). **And even then, most of them will**

**return, a few months or a year later, with swollen, painful, ulcerated, weeping legs**.

**Are there any specific points to be made about wound care in these unfortunate individuals?**

**In general, wound care in these patients should not differ from what we have discussed hitherto, except that everything becomes more difficult as the patient's bulk increases**. It is more difficult for the patient who often cannot access his own wounds, more difficult for his family, having to struggle with the dressings at home, and much more difficult for us in the wound care clinic. **Often, half of the encounter time is spent on positioning the patient to gain access to their wound**. And then we need help retracting the skin folds and elevating the limb, which is heavier than our assistant (■ Figure 19.1). Finally, you may need to crawl on the floor to debride the leg ulcer.

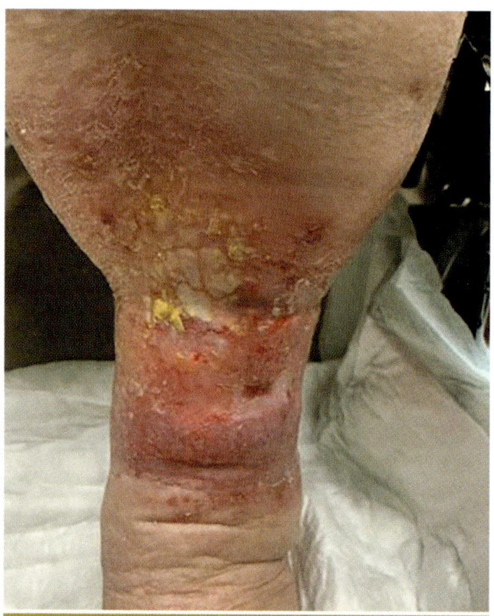

**Figure 19.1. Ankle stasis ulcer in a morbidly obese patient.**

[I did not want to include in this book (which is also aimed at the international reader) the complex topic of 'charging and reimbursement' for wound care in the USA, where what one earns is usually based on 'productivity' — on how many patients you see, and what you do with them. **But I want to mention only this, relating to the morbidly obese case**: for the average follow-up encounter for wound care, you are allowed to charge only for what you do, but not for the time and effort you invest. For example, for an encounter for a venous ulcer, you can charge either for debridement or for the Unna boot application — not both. Such a procedure in a 350-pound (158kg) patient may take three times as long as in a 'normal' patient. **Still, both are reimbursed the same.**]

**Otherwise, wound treatment is the same**. Except, you need more staff and wider wheelchairs; you need bariatric hoists (lifts) to prevent herniating your own lumbar discs. The wounds are deep and can be more productive — you need larger dressings and more material, which would be changed more frequently. **NPWT ('wound VAC') is commonly used in 'deep holes in the fat'**. Note that the subcutaneous layers in these patients are relatively poorly perfused. Thus, instead of using the typical pressure of -125mmHg, it is recommended to use lower pressures (-50 to -75mmHg) to preserve perfusion while still performing the healing task.

**And of course, optimal control of all the factors that prevent the wound from healing (➲ Chapter 3) is crucial.**

> **"Provide the morbidly obese patient with extra doses of respect and empathy — they need it!"**

# Chapter 20

## Miscellaneous wounds

*What's common is common, but don't miss the uncommon…*

These are the wounds which do not fall within the common entities detailed hitherto. They can also be termed 'atypical'. They are atypical because they can pop up spontaneously in atypical locations rather than the typical lower extremities, or pressure points. Also atypical may be their appearance and that they tend not to respond to prolonged conventional wound care.

In ➲ Chapter 2, I provided a long list of such rare and 'atypical' entities. A detailed discussion of each wound is beyond the scope of this brief monograph, but below are a few examples from my own experience to demonstrate how easy it is to miss the diagnosis.

I recall a middle-aged lady who was treated in our surgical outpatient clinic for a large non-healing wound in the groin. For many months, residents and attendings did not understand why such a clean-granulating wound was resistant to all balms and salves. Finally, I took a punch biopsy: it proved to be a poorly differentiated squamous cell carcinoma (SCC).

I recall a middle-aged truck driver with a 'scratch' on his cheek, which seemed to heal after a few weeks, only to recur a month later. He was given more 'wound care' until he was lost from follow-up, returning a year later with a large SCC invading his eye. He sued and was awarded $750,000. As I already mentioned (➲ Chapter 4), **chronic wounds that change appearance, progress, or are 'static' despite optimal care should be biopsied**.

Another case I remember is a young male patient with a non-healing skin ulcer on his leg. I excised it. Pathology reported 'non-specific' inflammation. He then presented to another hospital with multiple skin ulcers. Eventually, when he was diagnosed with **ulcerative colitis**, it became clear that the skin ulcers represented **pyoderma gangrenosum**, which typically develops in patients with inflammatory bowel disease. Excision should be avoided in such cases, as it can worsen or spread ulcers. Clearly, I missed the diagnosis! The patient sued but lost.

**"The message is this: as a wound care provider, you have to constantly look beyond the wound and see/assess the 'whole' patient. Yes, 'common things occur commonly'; 'think horses, not zebras' is a guiding principle in medicine, but sometimes the rare diagnosis is the correct one. You must think outside the box!"**

# Epilogue

Let me conclude this modest monograph with the commandments of wound care. People come up with 'ten commandments' for anything and everything these days — there are even '10 commandments of whiskey tasting'. And, of course, others have already come up with a list of 'commandments for wound care'. But here is my version of 13 commandments in the ■ Table below (please do not read it on Friday).

**The thirteen commandments of wound care.**

| Commandment | Comments |
|---|---|
| **1. Assess and treat the whole patient — look beyond the wound** | Define and address factors which would prevent/slow healing |
| **2. Establish the diagnosis** | Define/classify the cause of the wound |
| **3. Clean the wound** | Remove exudate, debris, etc. |
| **4. Debride the wound** | Remove/excise all non-viable tissues |
| **5. Address contamination and infection** | Choose local or systemic agents based on clinical and lab findings |

*Continued overleaf*

**The thirteen commandments of wound care *continued*.**

| Commandment | Comments |
|---|---|
| **6. Manage wound edges and the periwound** | Address callous, epibole, maceration, undermining |
| **7. Manage moisture balance** | Not too dry, not too wet |
| **8. Select the appropriate dressings** | Fit the dressing to the wound's characteristics |
| **9. Protect the wound and its surroundings** | Offloading... |
| **10. Reassess and change course if necessary** | Wound care is a dynamic process — the situation tends to change rapidly |
| **11. Avoid gimmicks and futile care** | You cannot heal everything but you can palliate |
| **12. Be kind and compassionate!** | These patients are often miserable — support and guide them |
| **13. Document everything, but don't exaggerate...** | Not only for the sake of 'big brother' but to allow the optimal continuation of care |

# Index


absorbent dressings 78
access to care 38
acetic acid 71
Alexander, Barry 75
alginate dressings 78
anaerobic culture 65–6
Angell, Marcia 118
Ankle-Brachial Index (ABI) 33–4, 88, 140–1
antibiotics 66–70
- intravenous 67
- ointments 68–9
- oral 67–8
- solutions 69–70
- susceptibility 61–2
- systemic 67–8
- topical 66, 68–70

anticoagulants 13–14, 27, 51, 100, 143
anti-rheumatoid drugs 27
antiseptics 70–1
Aquacel® 78
arterial ulcers *see* ischemic ulcers
assessment 29–43
- cultures 36–7
- documentation 39–43
- functional, psychosocial and system factors 37–8
- history-taking 30
- infection 34–6
- malignancy 38
- perfusion 33–4
- periwound 33
- sensation 34
- wounds 32–3

atheroemboli 143

autolytic debridement 49
autonomic neuropathy 128

Bacon, Francis 29
bacterial cellulitis 122, 123
bacteriology 57–9
bedsores *see* pressure ulcers
biofilm 25
biological debridement 48
blisters 162
'blue toe syndrome' 143
botulism 72
'bracelet effect' 18
burns 159–63
- blisters 162
- debridement 162
- dressings 162–3
- eschar 162
- first-degree 160, 162
- fourth-degree 160
- honey 163
- location 161
- major 162
- minor 161
- mixed degree 161
- moderate 161
- second-degree 160, 162–3
- silver-impregnated dressings 163
- silver sulfadiazine cream 162–3
- staging 160
- third-degree 160, 163
- total body surface area 161
- treatment 162–3

calciphylaxis 19
calf muscle pump 16
calluses 129, 133
capillary refill 140

cellulitis 122, 123
cephalexin 123
Charcot foot 130
chemotherapy drugs 27
clindamycin 69
*Clostridium botulinum* 72
coagulopathy 100
cognitive capacity 37
collagen dressings 80
collagenase-containing ointment 48–9
colonization 25, 35, 56–7
commandments of wound care 171–2
compliance 27, 37, 86–7, 112–13
compression 85–95
  compliance 86–7
  contraindications 88
  elastic (long stretch) 87
  graduated pressure 86
  importance of 85
  length of use 93–4
  maintenance 94–5
  non-elastic (short stretch) 87
  physiology 86
  practical points 93–4
  Profore® 89
  selection of system 86–7
  Setopress® 91–2
  Tubigrip® 92–3
  Unna boot 89
contamination 24–5, 35, 56–7
cooking metaphor of wound care 46
corticosteroids 27
cost of wound care 4
coumadin-induced skin necrosis 19
critical colonization 25
critical limb ischemia 140, 141, 142
cultures 36–7, 60–6, 130–1

debridement 47–53
  autolytic 49
  biological 48
  enzymatic 48–9
  mechanical 49
  non-selective 49, 51–2
  selective 49, 50–1
  surgical (sharp) 47, 49–52
decompensated heart failure 88
decubitus ulcers *see* pressure ulcers
dependency rubor 140
diabetic ulcers 11–12, 127–36
  calluses 129, 133
  Charcot foot 130
  clinical features 128–30
  cultures 130–1
  describing 129
  foot ischemia 130
  'football dressing' 133
  gangrene 131
  glycemic control 132
  immune deficiency 11, 128
  investigations 130–1
  management 132–3
  metabolic dysfunction 11, 128
  MRI 130
  negative pressure wound therapy 133
  offloading methods 132–3
  osteomyelitis 130
  pathophysiology 128
  peripheral neuropathy 11, 34, 128
  peripheral vascular disease 11, 128
  probe-to-bone test 129–30
  rate of healing 134
  recurrence prevention 134–5
  referral criteria 131
  salvage 135–6

surgical options 134
Toe-Brachial Index 130
X-rays 130
documentation 39–43
dressings 75–83
absorbent 78
advantages of modern dressings 76
alginates 78
Aquacol® 78
collagen 80
dry wounds 79–80
DuoDERM® 79
foam-based 78
frequency of change 82
hydrocolloids 79
hydrofiber 78
hydrogel 79
Mepilex® 78
moist wounds 78–9
moisture balance 77–8
occlusive 78–9
Opsite® 79
periwound 81–2
secondary 81–2
selection 77–80
silver-based 79–80
Silvercel® 78
soaking before removal 83
Tegaderm™ 79
transparent adhesive 79
wet wounds 78
wound bed preparation 82
Xeroform™ 79
drugs *see also* antibiotics
anticoagulants 13–14, 27, 51, 100, 143
coumarin (warfarin)-induced skin necrosis 19
wound healing 27

dry gangrene 131, 142
dry wounds 26
    dressings 79–80
DuoDERM® 79

edema 25–6, 122
elastic compression 87
electrical stimulation 117–18
elevation pallor 140
embolic skin ulcers 142–3
enzymatic debridement 48–9
epidermal advancement 21–2, 24
eschar 51, 99, 162
exudate 33

fistula 27
foam-based dressings 78
'football dressing' 133
foreign bodies 26
fucidic acid 69
functional factors 37–8

gangrene 131, 139, 142
gas emboli 71
gentamicin 69, 70
Gram stain 60–1

healing *see* wound healing
heart failure 88
heel fat pad 51
hematomas 13–14, 158–9
Hippocrates 77
history-taking 30
honey 71–2, 79, 109, 163
hydrocolloid dressings 79
hydrofiber dressings 78

hydrogel
- dressings 79
- injectables 116

hydrogen peroxide 70–1
hyperbaric oxygen therapy 117

immobility 16, 37, 145
immunosuppressants 27
infection
- bacteriology 57–9
- compression systems 88
- diagnosis and assessment 34–6, 55–6
- negative pressure wound therapy 99
- wound cultures 60–6
- wound healing 24–5

insect bites 19
intermittent claudication 137
intravenous antibiotics 67
ischemia
- critical limb ischemia 140, 141, 142
- 5Ps of limb ischemia 144
- negative pressure wound therapy 99
- wound healing 24

ischemic ulcers 12, 137–44
- Ankle-Brachial Index 140–1
- capillary refill 140
- clinical features 137–8
- compression 142
- dependency rubor 140
- diagnosis 140–1
- elevation pallor 140
- embolic skin ulcers 142–3
- examination 138–40
- gangrene 139, 142
- imaging 141
- intermittent claudication 137
- mixed type 137

peripheral pulses 139–40
'punched-out' nature 138
rest pain 138
treatment 141–2

Kalkum, Mathias 3

leg edema 25–6, 122
limb ischemia *see also* ischemic ulcers
critical 140, 141, 142
5Ps 144
negative pressure wound therapy 99
lipedema 17–18
lipodermatosclerosis 18–19
long stretch compression 87
lymphedema 16

maggots 48
malignancy 19, 38, 100
malignant transformation 19, 38
Marjolin's ulcer 38
measurement of wounds 32
mechanical debridement 49
Mepilex® 78
methicillin-resistant *Staphylococcus aureus* 59
metronidazole 69
MIC dilution 61
microbial continuum 25, 55
microemboli 143
mobility 16, 37, 145
moist wound dressings 78–9
moisture control 26, 77–8
mood 37
morbid obesity-related wounds 10, 15–18, 165–7
motor neuropathy 128
MRSA 59
mupirocin 69

necrobiosis lipoidica diabeticorum 19
necrotic tissue 24, 99
negative pressure wound therapy 97–103
  benefits 98
  candidates 98
  contraindications 99–100
  diabetic ulcers 133
  frequency of change 102
  'mini' system 102–3
  morbid obesity-related wounds 167
  patient considerations 100, 101–2
  periwound 100–1
  pressure ulcers 149–50
  prophylactic use 99
  SNAP™ 102–3
  sponge management 101
  system 97–8
  technical points 100–1
  terminating use 102
Nightingale, Florence 145, 150
non-compliance 27, 37, 86–7, 112–13
non-elastic compression 87
non-selective debridement 49, 51–2
non-steroidal anti-inflammatory drugs (NSAIDs) 27
nutritional deficiency 16–17

obesity 10, 15–18, 165–7
occlusive dressings 78–9
odor issues 109
offloading 132–3, 148, 151
Ogilvie, William Heneage 155
Opsite® 79
oral antibiotics 67–8
Osler, William 70
osteomyelitis 99, 130
oxygen delivery 28

packing wounds 52–3
palliative care 105–9
Paré, Ambroise 3
pentoxifylline 125
perfusion testing 33–4
peripheral arterial disease 88
peripheral neuropathy 11, 34, 128
peripheral pulses 33, 139–40
peripheral vascular disease 11, 128
periwound
    assessment 33
    dressings 81–2
    negative pressure wound therapy 100–1
placenta-derived products 116
polymorphonuclear cells 60
post-phlebitis syndrome 10
post-surgical wounds 12–13, 153–4
post-traumatic wounds 13–14, 155–9 *see also* burns
    hematomas 13–14, 158–9
    iatrogenic factors 156
    treatment 156
pressure injury 26, 37
pressure ulcers 12, 16, 145–51
    assessment 147–8
    common sites 145, 146
    medical device-related 146
    negative pressure wound therapy 149–50
    offloading 148, 151
    pathophysiology 145–6
    prevention 150–1
    stages 147, 148–9
    treatment 148–50
prevention 111–13
    diabetic ulcers 134–5
    pressure ulcers 150–1
    venous ulcers 125
probe-to-bone test 129–30

Profore® 89
*Pseudomonas spp.* 58, 67, 71
psychosocial factors 37–8
pyoderma gangrenosum 19, 170

qualitative wound culture 36
quality of care 27, 38
quantitative wound culture 36

radiation therapy 19, 27
rest pain 138

secondary dressings 81–2
selective debridement 49, 50–1
semiquantitative wound culture 36
sensation testing 34
sensory neuropathy 128
Setopress® 91–2
sharp debridement 47, 49–52
short stretch compression 87
silver-based products 71, 79–80, 163
silver sulfadiazine (SSD™) cream 69, 71, 162–3
Silvercel® 78
skin cancer 19, 38
skin fold maceration 16
skin grafting 125
SNAP™ 102–3
social-economic deprivation 27, 37–8
*Staphylococcus aureus* 58
    methicillin-resistant 59
stasis dermatitis 11, 122
Stomahesive® 101
surgery
    diabetic foot 134
    post-surgical wounds 12–13, 153–4
    surgical (sharp) debridement 47, 49–52
    venous ulcers 124–5

swabbing wounds 36–7
system factors 37–8
systemic antibiotics 67–8

Tegaderm™ 79
thirteen commandments of wound care 171–2
TIME 46
Toe-Brachial Index (TBI) 34, 130
topical antibiotics 66, 68–70
topical antiseptics 70–1
transparent adhesive dressings 79
trauma, repeated 26 *see also* post-traumatic wounds
triple antibiotic ointment 68–9
Tubigrip® 92–3

undermining 32
Unna boot 89

vacuum-assisted closure *see* negative pressure wound therapy
varicose veins 121, 122, 124
vasculitis 19
venous stasis 15
venous ulcers 10–11, 121–6
- cellulitis 122, 123
- clinical features 122
- compression therapy 123, 125
- diagnosis and investigations 122–3
- pathophysiology 121–2
- pentoxifylline 125
- rate of healing 123
- recurrence prevention 125
- skin grafting 125
- stasis dermatitis 11, 122
- surgical treatment 124–5
- varicose veins 121, 122, 124

warfarin-induced skin necrosis 19
wet gangrene 131, 142
wet wound dressings 78
wound care clinic, resources 5–6
wound care industry 3–5
wound cultures 36–7, 60–6, 130–1
wound debridement *see* debridement
wound healing 21–8
  adipose tissues 16
  external and iatrogenic factors 27–8
  mechanisms 21–2
  patient-related factors 23–4
  scoring systems 43
  wound-related factors 24–7
wound packing 52–3

Xeroform™ 79